Breathwork Exposed

What Works, What's Dangerous, and the Right Way to Breathe

By Dr. David Deppeler

Published by Kindle Direct Publishing

ISBN: 979-8-218-68407-5

Cover design by Anita Offerman | Editing by Amy White

Disclaimer: This book is for informational purposes only. It is not intended to serve as medical advice or to replace professional healthcare guidance. While every effort has been made to ensure accuracy, the author and publisher make no representations or warranties regarding the completeness, applicability, or reliability of the content provided. The breathing techniques described in this book are designed to support health and well-being but should be practiced responsibly. If you have any medical conditions, respiratory issues, or concerns about your health, consult with a qualified healthcare professional before implementing any new breathing practices. The author and publisher disclaim any liability for injuries or adverse effects resulting from the application of the information contained in this book.

For permissions, inquiries, or further information, contact: david@breatheyourtruth.com

Praise for *Breathwork Exposed*

"This book doesn't just teach you to breathe, it guides you back to the wisdom of your own body."

—Lee Holden, Qi Gong Master & Author of *Ready, Set, Slow!*

"David Deppeler brings clarity, nuance, and a refreshing dose of honesty to the world of breath training. His work integrates deep clinical insight with a practical, accessible style that makes the science usable whether you're an athlete, coach, or simply someone trying to breathe better. Through his contributions to *Oxygen Advantage*, particularly in the area of swimming and breathwork, David has helped push the field forward. *Breathwork Exposed* is a powerful, timely resource that strips away the hype and brings the focus back to what truly works."

—Patrick McKeown, Founder of Oxygen Advantage & Bestselling Author of *The Oxygen Advantage*

"Deppeler has cracked the code for breathwork and handed us an owner's manual. What he has been able to do with many of my professional runners is nothing short of profound. His work has helped my runners find more efficiency, durability, confidence and performance potential. This isn't wellness fluff, it's performance gold."

—David McHenry, PT & Performance Coach for Nike's Elite Runners

"This work is a game-changer. David and the *Breathe Your Truth* system helped me see how powerful breathwork is for recovery and performance without extra tech or cost. We were able to see some pretty immediate results and the BYT methods fit in seamlessly into our everyday training."

—Tim Brumlik, Under Armour 800m Coach

"I've always trained hard and paid attention to every variable, but a recurring side stitch kept showing up late in races and nothing seemed to fix it. Then I found *Breathe Your Truth*. David's approach helped me understand the deeper mechanics and chemistry of breath. Through his on-demand education, I retrained my system to breathe efficiently under pressure. I haven't had a side stitch since."

—Tristane Woodfine, Elite Canadian Marathoner

"David has been a trusted collaborator and knowledgeable educator in our yoga community for over 20 years. *Breathwork Exposed* beautifully blends breath science with the wisdom of yoga, challenging industry-wide misperceptions and opening the door to a more easeful, intelligent, embodied approach to yoga practice. This book is essential for anyone ready to breathe or teach with greater clarity and depth."

—SarahJoy Marsh, MA & Founder of *The Institute of Living Yoga*

"*Breathwork Exposed* brings coherence to the vast, often overwhelming world of breath practices, honoring their roots while offering clear, grounded guidance for modern seekers. This is a rare and valuable contribution to the evolving field of breath."

—Lee Lyon, author of *112 Meditations from the Book of Divine Wisdom*

Table of Contents

Foreword by Michael E. Long

Just between you and me, I don't read a book unless it's special. I certainly don't write a foreword. This is a great book, and I say that as someone who's written a few.

When I co-authored *The Molecule of More*, we came to realize that while any science book has to be backed up with the facts, it can't be boring. And any book about health has to deliver reproducible positive outcomes. David has done all those things.

In *Breathwork Exposed*, he has illuminated the practice of breathwork for the benefit of anyone who will slow down long enough to read it and act on it. Here's a lifetime of expertise presented in an engaging and practical way to make a difference in your physical health and your mental outlook. It's like hearing what you need to hear from a smart, compassionate friend.

Here's a guy who wants you to understand, wants you to find the improvement you seek, but who will not force it on you. Success comes only for those who take up the challenge themselves. Without your participation, all the help in the world counts for zip.

So this book is David rendered in ink, something like that. I know this because I've had the pleasure of working with him. He coached me on my own breathing and I saw the difference in my ability to calm myself, lower my heart rate, and get more benefit from my exercise. And that was just from the first ten minutes. I kid, but not much. What David teaches here gave me habits to feel better, which is quite an outcome when you thought things were peachy in the first place. This information created improvement where I didn't know any was due.

David's science-driven and compassionate approach to breathwork has one the highest ratios I've found of outcome-to-effort. Unlike the magic pills in TV ads and the click-your-heels-and-wish stuff so popular among otherwise intelligent people, breathwork is grounded in peer-reviewed research and a long, well documented history of remarkable results. I mention this because David has just as much contempt as I do for science-free promises. (See the introduction for his elegant fileting of breathwork charlatans and pay-me-please celebs.)

Turns out that changing the way you breathe can achieve something amazing.

Read on. You're about to feel better.

Michael E. Long
Co-author of *The Molecule of More*
Author of *Taming the Molecule of More*

Introduction

BREATHWORK IS EVERYWHERE, and it can be powerful. But don't be fooled. Not all breathing is created equal.

Tens of thousands of people believe that breathwork, especially "big breathing" taught by spiritual celebs, is a healthy habit. But the truth is it's *not* usually good for you. And the way you've been breathing up until now could be seriously compromising your health. Sorry to be the bearer of bad-breath news.

The fact that you're here makes me assume you're interested in breathwork and have probably come across some fancy techniques before. At the very least, deep breathing? But if you're a "pulmonaut" [1] (and a James Nestor fan) you may well have gone deeper. Maybe you've tried breathwork through the Wim Hof Method, the Breath of Fire, or the Holotropic approach? Yeah, me too. At one point, if it promised superhuman endurance, spiritual enlightenment, or an out-of-body experience, I was all in. The "weirder," the better. If someone told me hyperventilating upside down in an industrial freezer would unlock my full potential, I probably would have tried it, twice.

For those of you who have struggled with these practices, I've got some news for you: It's not your fault. The amount of flawed, overgeneralized breathing advice out there literally takes my breath away. Stick an undertrained yet lovable celebrity in a slick documentary, have them declare that the secret to ultimate health is gulping down air like a vacuum on overdrive, and boom, you've got a wellness disaster waiting to happen.

When breathing is manipulated without the right foundation, it can do us a lot more harm than good. As a Doctor of Science, I have this to say: if your body has told you to "stay away" from a breathwork session in the past by making you faint, or by making you light-headed, worried or sick, *start listening,* because you're probably doing something wrong for *your* body. Sorry you went through that.

For those of you who have loved the big breathing work and have felt full of boundless energy and inner peace, that's great. I have some extra information for you in this book that will make it even better, and even safer and healthier.

For now, know this: not all breathwork will serve you, no matter how sexy the marketing may be. Some methods can destabilize your nervous system, spike anxiety, and even reduce oxygen delivery to your cells. Over-breathing, despite what many claim, doesn't flood your body with extra oxygen. It does the opposite. It locks oxygen in the blood, making it harder for your cells to use it where it matters.

My goal with this book is to help you not only protect yourself in the fascinating yet very grey world of breathwork but also discover exactly what your body needs, tailored to you, based on real data you'll track along the way. Breathing isn't one-size-fits-all, and as you move through these pages, you'll learn how to measure, refine, and optimize your breath for your unique physiology and level of "breath fitness."

What Is Breathwork, Anyway?

Great question. It's one of those words that gets thrown around a lot, usually by someone sitting cross-legged in freshly ironed linen pants, telling you to "just breathe" followed by a lot of huffing and puffing and panpipes.

For the sake of linguistic accuracy, let's go straight to the source. According to the Cambridge English Dictionary, breathwork is "the practice of controlling your breathing in a particular way for physical or emotional benefits." [2]

In this book, I'll refer to breathwork as not just one practice, but an entire spectrum of practices, ranging from intentional over-breathing (hyperventilation techniques) to under-breathing (oxygen restriction training) to mindful breathing (observing slow, controlled breaths for relaxation and focus).

Most breathwork has a place somewhere, for someone. But the key is knowing when and how to use them properly. Otherwise, you're just rolling the dice with your nervous system, and let's just say, it doesn't always land in your favor.

Why You Should Read This Book

Apart from making my day and adding a couple of dollars into my bank account (thank you), there are other, more important reasons you should read this book. Mastering your breath for the better is one of the best things you can do for your health.

Think about it. Breathing is the first thing we do when we enter the world and the last thing we do before we leave it. In between, we do it about 20,000 times a day or more. [3] This means that any little thing we do incorrectly or correctly can have a significant impact on our life for better or worse. And yet, most of us never stop to notice how we're breathing.

With or without realizing it, we adopt unnatural breathing patterns that are just a little off and consequently make life harder for ourselves. But you already know how to breathe, and half of the time, healing is about learning how to get your mind out the way, so your body can do what it knows to do. This book's your chance to get back the wisdom you were born with.

If your breath has been working against you, you might be dealing with:

- Anxiety and chronic stress
- Chronic pain
- High blood pressure and an overactive nervous system
- Fatigue, brain fog, and poor recovery

- Sleep disturbances, snoring, or sleep apnea
- Stubborn injuries and muscle tension that never seem to go away
- Stagnant performance in fitness, sports, and daily life [3-8][9-12]

And here's the biggest myth we've been sold to make it all better: Breathe more!

Well, it won't. This book is going to show you why, for most of us, breathing *less* is actually better.

I don't mean to be a kooky breathwork kill-joy. Like I said, there can be a place for huffing and puffing, depending on the person. But I believe most of us lack the foundation to realize long term gains from these big breathing practices because we're not breathing well enough at rest.

Why Do I Care?

I didn't set out to become a breathwork guide, coach, specialist, or a pulmonary police officer. In fact, if you had told me years ago that I'd be writing a book on breathing, I would have laughed.

I was trained internationally in Orthopaedic Manual Physical Therapy, and I built my strait-laced career in the traditional clinic setting. I worked solely with people in pain, the new and the chronic. I was practicing at the top of my chosen profession it was all mostly… okay.

But despite all my training and hands-on experience in treating musculoskeletal conditions, I couldn't shake the feeling that something was missing. My work was mostly effective, but I sensed there was a deeper, more foundational way to help people beyond teaching them to move better.

The turning point came when I realised that breath was the missing link, an often-overlooked key that could amplify everything I was already doing. As I refined my approach, my patient base started to shift. More and more, I found myself working with elite athletes, Olympians, and high-performing professionals, all of whom had one surprising thing in common: their breathing patterns were holding them back.

What I once saw as a minor detail became impossible to ignore. Breathing dysfunction wasn't just an issue for people in pain; it showed up at every level of health and performance. And when we fixed it, the results were undeniable. Breathwork wasn't just a tool for recovery, it was a shortcut to unlocking someone's greatest potential.

In all transparency, my biggest learning came from making it though my own breathing problems. Like most of my patients, I had assumed breathing was automatic, something that just happened, something that couldn't get messed up by modern life. I was wrong.

My own breathwork journey started in a continuing education class 2005, with plastic canula tubes up my nose, staring at a capnography biofeedback screen. I was curiously watching real time data that showed me, plain as day, something was wildly off. My CO_2 levels were too low, my breathing was erratic, and my body was working harder than it needed to. It was validating, in a way. I had suspected something wasn't right with my health, and now I had proof. But what followed wasn't an instant breakthrough.

I now understood the general theory behind what was wrong, and what it would take to fix my breathing. I bought a capnography biofeedback device and got down to business. I tried all kinds of breathwork, and it wasn't long before everything I tried made my breathing worse. Small breaths, full breaths, fast breaths, slow breaths, breath holds. I tried to fix my breath the way I thought I had helped people fix their bodies all these years.

"You've got to put in the hard work, David," I told myself. "The more you work the more result you get." But there I was, armed with state-of-the-art technology and the best of intentions, pushing myself harder and harder… only to watch everything fall apart.

My numbers weren't improving; they were tanking, right alongside my sleep, my sense of well-being, and my mood. The harder I practised breathwork, the worse things got. Frustration doesn't even begin to cover it.

So, I did what any self-respecting clinician and scientist would do: I quit. I shoved the device into a closet, stopped obsessing, and got on with life. And then, something interesting happened. A few months later, out of the blue, my breathing felt… better. Smoother. Lighter. More natural. When I pulled out that same capnography device, the numbers confirmed what I already felt. My breathing had reset itself. My CO_2 levels were up, my breath rate had slowed, and, without force or over-analysis, I was breathing in a way that supported my body.

That moment changed everything. Twenty-plus years later, I'm still on track. I can tell when it's off, and I can get it back with little effort.

The solution to my breathing issues wasn't "big-breathing" breathwork, it wasn't forced breath holds, it was primarily getting out of my body's way and allowing its wisdom to take over. It was also about understanding how breathing works in real life, under real conditions, in a way that supports both the nervous system and physical function. But mostly, getting out of the way.

Newly passionate and inspired, I dove back into study. The science was there (though not widely used), as was the ancient wisdom to be found in things like Qi Gong, a centuries-old Chinese practice that combines gentle movement and meditation. As well as Yoga. The answers to my breathing puzzle were there all along.

As I started studying my patients' breathing patterns, high-level athletes, military personnel, CEOs, and everyday people trying to optimize their health, movement, and performance, I saw the same thing over and over again:

- People were breathing too much
- They were working too hard for too little gain
- Their nervous systems were wired for stress instead of calm

And the solution wasn't about holding their breath in frozen lakes. It was about doing the *right* breathwork, at the *right* time, in the *right* way for that *particular* patient.

At the risk of coming across as self-righteous, this approach is what separates real breath training from the flashy Instagram versions of breathwork that promise instant enlightenment and healing. Unlike many "breathwork instructors," I'm not here to sell you on exaggerated claims. I'm a clinician. My job is to help you understand the science, then give you a chance to get back to your healthiest "factory setting" breathing. Then you can leverage your breath to get more from the life you want to live, whether it's' training for an Olympic 800-meter run, enjoying a thoroughly nourishing walk in nature, or simply being able to engage a conversation without anxiety.

How Are We Going to Do That?

By now, it's probably obvious that this book will be a mix of good science, activities for you to try, and exposure to information informed by my experiences. At times, you'll be invited to entertain my crackpot evolving theories. But ultimately, this is a guide to breathing your truth with intention, progression, and measurable results.

You may be wondering how on earth we're going to do this via literature. That's a fair question.

And in all honesty, of course it would be preferable if we could work together face-to-face. But after doing this work for more than twenty years, I believe I can give you a framework to guide your journey in a book format. And it'll go something like this: Before you dive into the first chapter, I'll be including a snazzy QR code for you to scan. This will take you straight to an online tool to determine your Breath Fitness Score. I'll guide you through the entire thing using some easy-to-follow videos. This quick test will give you a measure of your current breathing fitness and resilience. It will give you a personal baseline to work with for the duration of this book.

As you go through the chapters, you'll end up learning ways to improve your breath efficiency to move that score forward. We'll also use your score to help identify the best version of a breathing practice. Remember, it's not a one-size fits all approach. With a little guidance from me, you're going to experiment, practice, and do all the right things to set you up for breathing success.

In a couple of months, you can retake the test to see how far you've come. Think of it as your before-and-after snapshot.

As a taster, here's what else we're diving into in *Breathwork Exposed*:

- The 5 Myths of Breathwork – The biggest misconceptions about breathing, why they persist, and what harm they may have done. Grr!

- The Triple M Triangle – A framework for breath mastery, covering Mechanics (how you breathe), Mix (your body's chemistry), and Mind (the breath's impact on your mental health)

- How to Build Your "Anxiety Shield" – Simple, safe breathing strategies to calm the nervous system and improve resilience

- Mouth Taping: Science or Hype? – The real effects of mouth taping for sleep, nasal breathing, and performance

- Breathing for Peak Performance – How to optimize breathwork for all kinds of exercise

Throughout the duration of this book, you'll have journey guideposts to assess, train, and learn from your breath. As a result, you'll get a stronger body, sharper mind, and greater control over your health and performance now and in the future.

Ready?

Then let's begin.

Activity 1: Get Your Breath Fitness Score

Before we start fine-tuning your breath, let's figure out where you stand right now. Knowing where you are gets you closer to your inner wisdom, which is an infinitely stronger guide than me and even this fantastic book.

That's the spirit in which I've developed the Breath Fitness Score Calculator, a simple but effective tool to provide a window into your breathing efficiency so you can track your progress over time.

For the wise researcher in you: As of 2025, this tool has yet to be completely scientifically validated. I've grabbed the available science and combined it with the clinical experience of the Breathe Your Truth team. It's our best shot right now, and we'll keep the door open for upgrades based on emerging evidence.

For the wise researcher in you: As of 2025, this tool has yet to be completely scientifically validated. I've grabbed the available science and combined it with the clinical experience of the Breathe Your Truth team. It's our best shot right now, and we'll keep the door open for upgrades based on emerging evidence. Take the test by scanning the QR code and completing the activities.

Alternatively, you can go straight to breatheyourtruth.com/score. You'll then receive your results and find out where your breath stands today. After you have your results, you should:

- Write it down or take a screenshot. This is your starting point
- Check in every few weeks and retake the test to see how you're improving
- Aim for at least a four-point improvement after a few weeks. That's a clinically significant shift, but any positive change you sense is a win

Will this tool help you become an enlightened being of breathing, leading to levitation and immortality? Probably not. But I can tell you this for sure: it's going to give you a starting point to vastly improve your health, and hey, maybe even your life.

And, drumroll, please...

You'll have the proof to back it up.

Chapter 1:
The 5 Big Breathing Myths, Busted

LET'S START WITH THE BOMBSHELL: Most people have messed up their breathing.

I know. It sounds ridiculous. You've been breathing your whole life, and last time you checked, you're still here. So, what's the problem?

First off, breathing is both automatic *and* under your control. And thanks to modern life, most of us have unknowingly micromanaged our breath into dysfunction. In other words, we've made something that should be effortless... a struggle, without even realizing it.

Right now, your breathing might be working *against* you, kind of like running with untied shoelaces and wondering why you keep face-planting. And if bad breathing habits weren't enough, the modern breathwork industry, with all due respect, has turned breathing into something of a circus.

We've got self-proclaimed "gurus" preaching that *more* breathing equals limitless energy. We've got viral trends pushing hyperventilation until you have in intimate relationship with your spirit animal. And then there's Wim Hof, the Iceman himself, shouting: "Breathe, motherf*cker, breathe!" while throwing himself into a frozen lake. Some followers have managed to get themselves in serious physical danger. A few have even died. (Not saying it's all Hof's fault, by the way, but still.)

These practices can be the perfect recipe for a binge-worthy Netflix documentary (or five), but clinically? It's a mess. And yet, buried in all the hype, there are truths on both ends of the spectrum, from big breathing to gentle mindfulness.

Before we dive into what actually works, let's clear up what doesn't. Here are the five biggest myths about breathing – the ones that are keeping people stuck, tired, and (ironically) gasping for air.

Myth 1: More Is Better

If you've read James Nestor's *Breath: The New Science of a Lost Art* or Patrick McKeown's *The Oxygen Advantage*, [1, 13] you probably already suspect where this is going. If you haven't, buckle up – this is going to challenge everything you thought you knew about breathing.

Here's the first truth: More breathing does not mean more oxygen. It sounds counterintuitive because you'd think that inhaling more would automatically flood your body with it, giving you more health and spiritual tranquillity. But that's not how it works. In fact, for most people, most of the time, breathing more actually means getting *less* oxygen where it matters.

Oxygen is fuel, but simply breathing more doesn't deliver more of that fuel to your cells. Instead, it disrupts your blood chemistry and traps oxygen in your bloodstream rather than releasing it into your tissues. The result? Your cells get *less* oxygen. And when your cells get less oxygen, that means less energy, slower recovery, and a body that's working harder than it needs to. It's like filling up your car with fuel but forgetting to turn the key. The oxygen is there, but it's not making it where it needs to go.

Instead of feeling energized, healed and focused, like you were promised by your guru of choice, you may end up fatigued, light-headed, foggy, anxious, ungrounded or tense. And you don't even realise that your breathing is the culprit.

The vast majority of us breathe too much in general, especially at rest, which is ironic because over-breathing makes resting (and everything else) so much trickier.

Right about now, you might be thinking, *This probably isn't my story. I don't breathe too much! I actually find myself holding my breath.*

I hate to break it to you, but that's actually one of the biggest signs of over-breathing. You're noticing the breath-holding part, but what you don't notice is that just before that, you were probably inhaling like a maniac, over-breathing without realizing it, until your body hit the brakes and exasperated, screamed at you, "Hey, would you quit breathing so much!?"

And this is not just anecdotal: research backs this up. Researcher Dr. Kyle Kiesel found that 60-80% of people over-breathe to the extent that it impairs their functional movement. [14, 15] In addition, decades of medical records compiled by Dr. Rakhimov (a Russian Buteyko researcher and instructor) show that modern humans are breathing more (and breathing worse) than ever before. [16]

Another interesting observation is that bad breathing happens most while we're chilling. Which is why so many people feel constantly on edge. Exercise, ironically, is the one time we tend to breathe more efficiently because movement helps regulate breath rate and blood chemistry. But when we're sitting at our desks, scrolling through our phones, or trying to fall asleep? That's when we're at our worst.

Why are we doing this? Why are we breathing too much to our own detriment? In all honesty, I don't completely know how to answer that question. But I do have some theories. It more than likely has to do with a combination of the way modern humans move (or don't move), the way we process stress, and the way we're told to breathe by the mainstream. And of course, the general state of our mental health.

Let's continue the geek-fest and move onto the second myth, which further explains why breathing more isn't such a good idea.

Myth 2: CO_2 Is the Bad Guy

We've been conditioned to think of carbon dioxide (CO_2) as the villain, the waste product of respiration, the thing we need to exhale and get rid of as quickly as possible. It's the gas that gets blamed for everything from climate change to soda-induced burps.

But carbon dioxide isn't some toxic byproduct that needs to be expelled at all costs. When it comes to your body, carbon dioxide is a VIP in maintaining your blood's acid-base balance. Without it, your pH would be all over the place and you'd feel… well, terrible.

Your blood operates within a very specific pH range (about 7.35-7.45) [17] and too far in either direction, you're in trouble. When your cells do their thing (burning fuel for energy) they produce CO_2 as a byproduct. Instead of just floating around uselessly, CO_2 dissolves in your blood and forms carbonic acid (H_2CO_3). This acid quickly breaks down into bicarbonate (HCO_3^-) and hydrogen ions (H^+), which help regulate your body's pH balance. If things get too acidic, bicarbonate soaks up those extra hydrogen ions like a biochemical sponge. Too alkaline? The system reverses, releasing H^+ to bring balance back. [6, 18-22] In other words, CO_2 is vital and non-negotiable to keep your body's pH balance healthy.

When you over breathe and CO_2 levels drop, your blood vessels constrict, making it harder for oxygen to reach your brain, muscles, and organs. That means oxygen gets trapped in the blood instead of getting delivered where it's needed. The result? Fatigue, brain fog, poor circulation, and even a weaker immune system. It's like making every system in your body work twice as hard just to keep up. Over time, this can lead to chronic stress, inflammation, and reduced efficiency in everything from digestion to recovery.

For the mad scientists among you, this is called the Bohr Effect, and it's a fundamental principle of human physiology. Discovered by Danish scientist Christian Bohr in 1904, this effect explains that oxygen is only optimally released from red blood cells when CO_2 levels are at a healthy level, i.e., when you're NOT over breathing. [23]

Moral of the story? Don't hate on CO_2; it's literally keeping you alive.

Myth 3: You Can Huff and Puff Your Way to Enlightenment

Many of today's sexy breathwork techniques are built on the idea that by breathing in extreme ways, you can access altered states, unlock hidden potential, or even connect with the divine. Hyperventilate just right, and you might just see the face of God, uncover your life's purpose, or transcend the need to pay taxes.

Now, I'm not here to bash these techniques. I've tried them. I've had fascinating experiences with them and enjoyed the natural highs. But here's what's not being said enough: most people are not ready for these kinds of breathing techniques, mechanically nor neurologically. In other words, most people will just get really dizzy, possibly have a novel transient experience, or maybe just pass out.

Breathing in extreme ways, whether it's intentional over-breathing (hyperventilation) or oxygen restriction (hypoxia), isn't inherently bad in small doses for those who have excellent breath fitness scores. These activities have a time, a place, and a physiological impact. But done without proper preparation, I have seen them lead to:

- Panic attacks
- Blackouts
- Overloaded nervous system responses
- Reinforced chronic breathing pattern dysfunction
- Generalized anxiety

Amongst other things.

Now, let's talk about God. Why do so many people claim that breathwork connects them to the divine? Why do some say it feels just as powerful as psychedelics like ayahuasca or magic mushrooms?

The answer lies in hormones and neurotransmitters. During an intense breathwork session, your body floods with adrenaline, endorphins, and altered oxygen levels that can create a temporary feeling of euphoria or transcendence. This is real chemistry at work. It's in a similar playing field to runner's highs, deep meditation states, or the effects of plant medicines and other recreational drugs.

Now, is that such a terrible thing? Not necessarily. Feeling connected, inspired, or spiritually awake through your breathing alone can be a wonderful experience. But here's the issue: feeling good doesn't always mean being *healthy*.

Think of it like this: eating chocolate muffins on a Friday night feels amazing. That warm, gooey goodness? Instant joy (at least for me). But just because it *feels* good doesn't mean it *is* good for you. It's not supporting your health long-term. Breathwork is the same. Just because a session makes you feel closer to God doesn't mean it's true. Sorry.

Here's the bottom line: if big breathing breathwork is your thing, great. If you're using it in moderation to explore consciousness and spirituality, fine. But it should never come at the cost of your nervous system, blood pH, sanity, or your general health. Use your Breath Fitness Score, or some other metric (a few more to come), to track the effects of this kind of breathwork over time.

Myth 4: 10 Deep Breaths Will Make You Feel Better

Ah, the classic.

It's what people say when you're stressed, frustrated, or one email away from quitting your job and moving to a remote island. I'd bet you've even given that piece of advice to a loved one yourself.

It's not all wrong, but the way we often use it is... very wrong. You see, if we just took one, well-distributed breath using our diaphragm, that would be helpful. But instead, we overdo it. We take many big, deep breaths, convinced that more must be better. Enter the fourth most popular (and equally flawed) recommendation: "Take ten deep breaths."

No! DO NOT TAKE TEN DEEP BREATHS when you're already teetering on the edge of anxiety. That's like throwing gasoline on a fire and wondering why it won't go out. One big breath? Fine. Ten in a row? Now you're hyperventilating your way into feeling worse.

If you're putting the pieces together, you'll see the issue here. That one big deep breath can feel great: it stretches your muscles, opens up your chest, and maybe even comes with a satisfying sigh. So yes, take ONE and enjoy the feeling. It's good. But don't tank your CO_2 levels by taking it too far and sending your nervous system into chaos.

Instead of continuing to gulp in air like a fish on land, transition into light, low, and slow breathing after ONE big breath. This restores your CO_2 balance and actually helps you feel better.

Side note: Most of us have also been conditioned to think "deep" means "big." That's a problem. When people take a so-called "deep" breath, they usually inhale as much air as possible, lifting their chest, expanding their ribs, and making themselves feel momentarily larger. But now you know they're flooding their system with more air, not more oxygen, all while depleting their CO_2 levels.

Proper deep breathing isn't about volume – it's about location. Instead of thinking about taking in more air, think about sending your breath lower into your diaphragm rather than your chest. Instead of repeatedly inhaling forcefully, breathe low and slow, allowing your belly to expand while your shoulders stay still.

That's the kind of deep breathing that actually calms your nervous system, improves oxygen delivery, and does what people expect a "deep breath" to do.

Myth 5: The More You Work on Your Breath, the Better It Gets

The moment we focus on our breath, we often get in our own way.

We start trying too hard, taking bigger, slower, or more controlled breaths than necessary, second-guessing every inhale and exhale, and turning what should be an effortless process into a mental obstacle course. Instead of helping, this overcorrection often disrupts our natural rhythms, making breathing feel forced, unnatural, or even stressful for some people.

Time and time again, capnography devices (biofeedback tools that reveal CO_2 levels in real time) show us the same thing. The moment people start focusing on their breath, their breathing patterns actually get worse at first. It's like trying to perfect your walking technique: suddenly, something automatic feels awkward and clunky just because you're thinking about it too much.

You might have noticed the irony here. You picked up this book expecting to improve your breathing. You took the time to complete a test, got a breathing score, and now you're probably thinking you wasted your money. You didn't. You still need to change your breathing, but instead of forcing it, we'll nudge it.

Before we move forward, let's try something simple so you can experience this firsthand. Right now, without altering anything, just pay attention to your breath.

- Where do you feel it?
- Is it in your chest, belly, or somewhere else?
- Are you breathing through your nose or mouth?
- Is it fast, slow, shallow, deep?

Most people, when they do this, immediately start breathing differently. That's normal. But over the next few days, I want you to keep noticing your breath in different situations: when you're stressed, when you're relaxed, when you're exercising, and when you're about to fall asleep, *without* trying to fix it.

Because before we can fix anything, we have to understand what's happening.

What's Next?

Now that we've tackled the biggest myths about breathing, we can start getting into how to actually breathe better.

In the upcoming three chapters, we'll explore the three pillars of breathwork: The Mechanics, the Mix, and the Mind, also known as the Triple M. And we'll go over how to bring them into balance for better health, energy, and performance.

Chapter 2:
Welcome to the Mechanics Lab

WHAT IF I TOLD YOU THAT 90% of all athletes show signs of poor breathing? [24] That should be interesting to you. Why? Because if the best performing humans on Earth are struggling, what does that mean for the rest of us?

Under pressure, whether it's during exercise, stress, or deep focus, we're all vulnerable to compromised and inefficient breathing. And this connects directly to some of the most pressing issues of our time: the skyrocketing rates of anxiety, depression, cardiac issues, and gut dysfunction. All of these have been shown, in various ways, to link back to breathing. When the breath is off, our entire system pays the price.

But what if, instead of falling apart under pressure, your breathing actually supported you? That's what we're here to explore. And to do that, we're going to break breathing down into its three fundamental components so we can understand it all better.

I call this the Triple M:

- Mechanics (how we breathe)
- Mix (what happens inside our blood)

- Mind (how breath influences stress, focus, and performance)

We'll cover them separately, but they are inseparable in practice.

Improve one, and the others follow. Master all three, and you'll revolutionize the way your body moves, performs, and recovers. Let's dive into the first M.

Mechanics 1.0: How Your Body *Really* Wants to Breathe

Let's get this mechanics party started with a fact: breathing isn't just breathing. Not as you know it, anyway. What I mean to say is that what we refer to as "breathing" is not one single process. It's actually three totally separate but connected systems working together. There's "breathing," "respiration" and "gas transport."

Here's how the three processes work in your body:

- Breathing: This is the physical act of moving air in and out of your lungs using your nose, mouth, diaphragm, rib cage, back, chest and other breathing muscles. All of these are part of your breathing mechanics, the physical parts that make breathing possible. You can think of breathing as ventilation – when your body brings air in and pushes it out. This can be both conscious and unconscious.

Breathing happens when you try, and it still keeps happening when you don't. Thank goodness!

- Respiration: The second process happens on a cellular level. Once air reaches your lungs, oxygen is transferred into your bloodstream and delivered to your cells. There, it fuels energy production, and in the process, creates carbon dioxide as waste. You don't control this part. It's unconscious.

- Gas Transport: This is the system that actually does the "moving" of oxygen from your lungs into your bloodstream and shuttles carbon dioxide out of your body. Again, you don't have conscious control over this part.

Why am I telling you this? Because I'm exposing you to where the real "problem" lies.

Of the three processes, the first one (breathing) is probably the real culprit when things go wrong. The second two steps (respiration and gas transport) are automatic and handled by your body without your input. But breathing? That's where we have control, and where we have the opportunity to mess it all up.

Your body is incredibly good at respiration (using oxygen in your cells) and gas transport (moving oxygen and carbon dioxide through the bloodstream). But it can only work with the air you bring in. If the way you're physically inhaling and exhaling is inefficient, your body doesn't get the oxygen it needs, forcing it to compensate in ways that can leave you feeling sluggish, anxious, or short of breath.

When you optimize *how* you breathe, i.e., the mechanics, your entire system works better. And of course, if we don't, that's when things can get ugly.

When Breathing Goes Very Wrong

Pain is your body's alarm system, and when it starts screaming (low back pain, neck tension, that stubborn knot between your shoulder blades that no massage ever fully fixes?) it's trying to tell you something.

Both research and my clinical experience keep saying the same thing: sometimes, chronic pain is caused by nothing other than dysfunctional breathing patterns. Especially pain directly linked to the neck, shoulders, and low back.

Why? When your breath is stuck high in the chest, fast, shallow, and tight, your neck and shoulder muscles start overworking. They try to help you breathe because the diaphragm isn't doing its job. Over time, they tighten up and become weak from chronic overuse.

If you're slouching, your ribs compress, making it even harder for the diaphragm to work properly. The breath gets even shallower, and the cycle continues.

And if your diaphragm isn't working as it should, your lower back can start to hurt. The diaphragm is anchored into the lumbar spine. So, if it's not moving well, you lose the subtle stabilizing pressure that supports your spine, forcing your lower back to compensate. You can stretch all day long, but if your breathing is dysfunctional, the pain will keep coming back. So, it's worth taking a look at your breathing mechanics.

Breath Battles and Breakthroughs

We don't think much about breathing until it betrays us. One minute, you're cruising. The next you're gasping at the top of the stairs, fighting for air mid-swim, or hunched over with a side stitch that just won't quit.

Let me introduce you to three people who thought they were stuck with their limitations, until they changed their breathing mechanics.

Todd's Story: The Breathless Swimmer

Todd, a retired tech executive turned triathlon devotee, had put in the work. After a year of swimming drills and hours of expert coaching, he should've been gliding through the pool with ease.

But after just one lap? He was gassed. It didn't make sense. He was strong on the bike. Solid on the run. His swim technique coach swore he was doing everything right. But the second he hit the water; it was like someone pulled the air plug. His issue was classic.

It was because on land, Todd was stuck in an upper chest breathing pattern. Every inhale sent his collarbones sky-high, while his belly stayed motionless. Even when prompted to "breathe low," nothing changed. His diaphragm was playing half the game it should.

Worse yet, he had little control over his exhale. Air just fell out of him. His body had learned to scrape by on land, but in water, where breath control is non-negotiable, his system panicked. His nervous system, sensing a lack of control, overreacted, sending his heart rate skyrocketing and his endurance plummeting.

Before Todd could master breathing in the pool, he had to optimize his mechanics on land by retraining the diaphragm so he could breathe low and deep. Once that clicked? Not only did swimming feel smoother, his cycling and running levels jumped up a notch too.

Janice's Story: The Scale of the Stairs

Janice was no slouch. A retired education director, she was used to leading meetings, juggling responsibilities, and running a tight ship. She walked daily, did Pilates twice a week, and still had more energy than most twenty-somethings.

Except... on the stairs. Two flights up to her apartment, and she'd hit the door panting.

"I walk at least ten thousand steps every day," she said. "Why do two flights feel like Everest?"

We started digging. Allergies? Check. Constant congestion? Yep. Years of mouth breathing? You bet.

Due to suboptimal mechanics, Janice's diaphragm had gone on vacation. Her neck and chest muscles had taken over the workload, and they were exhausted.

She described it perfectly one day: "I feel like I'm breathing from my collarbones."

We went back to basics. First up: building nasal breathing tolerance. At first, it felt weird. She'd get that panicky "there's not enough air!" feeling. But with slow, patient work, starting with easy walks and sitting practice, her nose started to feel less like a straw and more like an open gate.

Then came diaphragm training. Learning how to feel the breath in her belly, sides, and back, not just her chest. Little by little, she started to trust it.

A couple of months later, I got a text from her:

"The stairs aren't a big deal anymore. I barely notice them. I think my diaphragm's back from vacation."

I texted back: "Tell it I said welcome home."

Tristane's Story: The Marathon Runner with Side-Stitch

Tristane Woodfine, a Canadian marathon runner, reached out after having to drop out of yet another race. The cause? A side stitch (that sharp, nagging pain that feels like someone's jabbing a knife under your ribs). He told me he could tolerate nose breathing for the first few miles, but after that? Game over.

A little education, consistent work non his mechanics, and two months later? Side stitch, gone. The fix wasn't some massive overhaul. Instead, Tristane made a few small but powerful tweaks: he warmed up and cooled down slower and more intentionally, he built up his tolerance to nasal breathing, and most importantly, he slowed down his breathing at the start of every run.

This woke up his diaphragm, and this alone helped Tristane break the cycle. His body stopped rebelling, the pain disappeared, and his personal best times followed soon after.

It's wild how many positive changes you can make by fixing your breathing mechanics. Stuff that used to feel like "just how it is" (chronic pain, fatigue, side stitches) often vanish into thin air.

The 3 Mechanical Tweaks for Better Breathing

Now that we've established *you* are the problem (acceptance is step one), let's talk about how to fix it.

The next three mechanical ingredients will help you do more than just breathe; they'll enhance your endurance and performance, whether you're training for a marathon or simply want to climb a flight of stairs without gasping. They'll also improve how oxygen is delivered to your cells, so your body actually makes use of the air you inhale. And they support your nervous system, which means better sleep, lower stress, and sharper mental focus.

The best part? None of this is overly complex, and you can start training your mechanics right away. Half the game is simply returning to your body's "factory settings" and letting your body do what it was designed to do.

Secret Ingredient 1: Nose Breathing

Closing your mouth when you breathe is a game-changer. As well as building your CO_2 tolerance, nasal breathing:

- Filters, warms, and humidifies air for smoother respiration
- Encourages proper diaphragm engagement, setting the foundation for good breath mechanics
- Produces nitric oxide, which boosts circulation and oxygen absorption [25-32]

If breathing through your nose doesn't feel easy at first, that's a sign your airway is a little out of shape. You've built a habit of mouth-breathing more than you think, but that's okay. You're not alone. Stick with it. Your body will adapt, and the benefits will be amazing.

As you keep reading, try breathing through your nose mindfully. You don't need to take longer or bigger breaths. Just breathe low, light, and easy.

And if you're a nighttime mouth breather, no worries. I've got a whole section coming up just for you.

Secret Ingredient 2: Belly Breathing (Done Right)

People say, "Always breathe into your belly," but let's be clear; your lungs are not in your belly.

What we actually mean by "belly breathing" is 360-degree breath expansion where your breath moves freely through your belly, ribs, and back... in all directions. That's the gold standard.

To get there, you need to learn to use that large, dome-shaped muscle I mentioned earlier: your diaphragm. Think of your diaphragm like a fleshy jellyfish, expanding and contracting in rhythmic waves. When you inhale, the diaphragm contracts and flattens, pressing down on your internal organs. That downward motion builds positive pressure in your belly and creates negative pressure in your chest, just enough suction to draw air into your lungs.

It's not about forcing air in; your diaphragm is making space for it. Like a piston pulling downward, it gives your lungs room to expand. On the exhale, the diaphragm relaxes and domes back up, and the air flows out naturally.

When it functions properly, it doesn't just help you breathe; it transforms the way your entire body operates, including but not limited to stabilizing your spine, improving your posture, boosting digestion, improving circulation and optimizing your nervous system. [6, 24, 30, 33-46]

Want to introduce yourself to this amazing muscle? Let's try belly breathing, using the diaphragm, now.

- Rest the tip of your tongue gently on the roof of your mouth (this helps to unclench your jaw)
- Place your hand just below your belly button
- Breathe through your nose, sending the air all the way to the bottoms of your lungs (imagine the air traveling down into your hips)
- As your lower lungs fill, allow your belly to move out, your ribs to separate and your back to expand
- Feel that first movement in your belly? That's your diaphragm in action!

Tadah. For now, don't worry about getting it "right." If it felt clunky, you may be a little out of practice and that's okay. Just keep experimenting with sending your breath a bit lower into your belly, letting your jellyfish inflate.

If this process takes a while to master, welcome to the club. Most people have been unknowingly holding tension or underusing their diaphragm for years. Which brings us to the next ingredient...

Secret Ingredient 3: Softness: Drop the Tension

Most of us have unknowingly trained ourselves to hold tension in key areas of the body that should be soft and responsive. When this happens, simply put, the diaphragm gets blocked and can't work its magic. The breath becomes restricted, shallow, and inefficient. It's like trying to run a marathon while clenching your legs the entire time; it's completely unnecessary and exhausting.

There are four areas of tension that sabotage smooth, soft, natural breathing with the diaphragm:

- Pelvic Floor: If your pelvic floor is constantly tight (which is more common than you'd think), it restricts the movement of the diaphragm, preventing full breath expansion.

- Chest: Stress and emotional tension tend to live in the upper chest. This keeps the ribs tight and the breath trapped in a small, shallow zone. This feels like your lungs are stuck in a breath prison.

- Mid-Back: The area between the shoulder blades tends to tighten up and get weak due to bad posture and screen time. This stiffness limits the ability of the ribs to expand fully, cutting off the movement of the diaphragm and a huge part of your breathing potential.

- Jaw/Face: Clenching the jaw or furrowing the brow sends a subconscious signal to your nervous system that you're in fight-or-flight mode, keeping the whole body on high alert. This tension keeps breathing shallow too.

The fix? Learn to let go.

When you do, your breath drops lower, slows down, and moves more easily. Instead of forcing better breathing, think of it like clearing the path. Try this right now: Unclench your jaw. Soften your shoulders. Take an easy breath in through your nose and let it drop into your belly.

Feel that? A little more ease? That's the softness you want.

Integrate What You Just Learned

Now let's be real. If I tell you that you need to carve out extra time every single day for a dedicated breath practice session, you won't. At best, it'd last for a few days, then you'd fall off the bandwagon, because you're a human being. And honestly, I don't blame you.

The good news is that you don't have to create a time-consuming new routine. Over and over, I see people make real, lasting progress by simply doing better with the things they're already doing. No extra hours.

But if you'd like somewhere to begin, a framework, here is what I recommend to my clients:

Step 1: Reset Your Breath in Stillness

Before you integrate better breathing into movement, start with stillness. Sitting is the least physically demanding way to repattern your breath. Just a minute of focused awareness first thing in the morning can work wonders.

- Bring your attention to your lower abdomen or ribcage
- Notice how your breath naturally drops when you focus on it. No forcing
- Feel the movement, allowing it to be smooth, steady, and effortless
- Enjoy the calming effect of nasal breathing for as long as time allows

Step 2: Link Breath Awareness to Daily Habits

To make this stick, tie your breath awareness to things you already do. This is called "habit stacking." You could do this:

- Before and after meals. Drop into slow, low breathing to aid digestion

- While reading, working, or playing computer games. Use these moments to check in on how low, light and slow your breath can go
- Every time you reach for your phone. Instead of doom-scrolling straight away, take one good breath first. Then pay attention to your breathing while you scroll
- During conversations. When listening, soften your body and breathe a little more smoothly

Step 3: Breath Training While Moving

Stillness builds the foundation, but life isn't still. That's why the next step is learning to breathe well while moving. Later in this book, we'll dive into specific breathwork strategies for exercise, whether you're lifting weights, running, swimming, doing yoga, or practising Qi Gong.

For now, let's keep it simple. During low-intensity activities like walking, stretching, or even doing household chores, stick to the fundamentals from this chapter: breathe through your nose, breathe low into the belly using your diaphragm, and keep your breath calm and light. Less air, not more.

If your breath suddenly shifts to your chest or slips out through your mouth, take it as feedback. That's your signal to slow down, soften the effort, and let your breath drop lower and smoother again.

Final Thoughts on Mechanics

Phew. You've just taken a deep dive into the crazy world of breathing mechanics. And if you're still here, I hope something's clicking.

You've seen that great breathing isn't some rare talent or mystical gift. It's trainable. It's doable. And it starts with awareness.

When your mechanics are dialled in, everything improves: posture, energy, sleep, movement, even mood. You now know the secret isn't to breathe more, but to breathe better. To stop fighting your breath and start working with it.

You've seen how poor mechanics can lead to pain, tension, fatigue, and stress. You've also learned that small shifts like using your nose and diaphragm more and letting go of tension can create a ripple effect that changes how you feel in your body.

And this is just the beginning. There's so much more ahead. You're building a skill that will serve you in every part of life. Let's keep going.

Activity 2: Wake Up Your Diaphragm

Want to go a bit deeper to put this into practice? Try this short Qi Gong routine designed to gently wake up your diaphragm and reinforce your learning. Go to breatheyourtruth.com/breathwork-exposed or scan the QR code:

Now, if you're thinking, "Wait...Qi what?" Let me explain.

Qi Gong (pronounced "chee-gong") is an ancient Chinese system of coordinated movement, breathing, and awareness. The phrase loosely translates as "the art of cultivating vital energy," or, more to the point for our purposes, "how to move and breathe in a way that prevents disease before it even starts." Not bad, right?

Qi Gong is like the forgotten sibling of Yoga, but just as powerful. It's been used for centuries to calm the mind, balance the breath, and train the body to respond, rather than react, to stress. And it's shockingly good at helping people unlearn dysfunctional breathing habits.

Chapter 3:
The Mix of Breathing (Where the Devil Hangs Out in the Details)

NOW, I KNOW I JUST TOLD YOU that crappy breathing mechanics are usually the culprit behind most breath-related issues. That's still true. But every now and then, everything *looks* great from the outside. The posture's dialed. The breath is low and slow. But something's still… off.

Although you're nose-breathing and using your diaphragm, the amount of air you're pulling in may be too much. The breath is just a little too big. Or a touch too frequent. Nothing dramatic. But it's enough to push you over the line into hyperventilation. That's where the devil hides, in the details.

It's like driving a car that veers one degree to the right. You don't notice it at first… but thirty miles later, you're in a ditch wondering what happened. That tiny drift chips away at your CO_2 levels, messes with oxygen delivery, and pulls your whole Mix off balance.

When I say "Mix," I'm talking about the second M, the biochemistry that comes after breathing. The respiration part that comes after the Mechanics.

This part of respiration is the glue that turns good mechanics into great results. And it drops straight into the middle of your day, your mood, your focus, your performance. You'll see how just a few tweaks in how you support your chemistry can shift everything from energy to emotional resilience. That's the magic (and mischief) of chemistry.

Sara's Story: Perfect Mechanics, Rogue Mix

Sara is one of those people who radiates good vibes. A well-known Yoga instructor, loved by her students, and, from the outside, someone who had breathwork dialed in. But one day, after class, she confided something in me.

"I can't do many of the breath practices I teach without getting a headache. It used to happen once in a while... now it's almost every class. Do you think I could be doing something wrong with the way I breathe?"

Yes. Yes, I did. We took a look. As you'd expect from someone with years of Yoga under her belt, her breath mechanics looked beautiful at first glance. Smooth. Controlled. Good diaphragm activity, great lung capacity, flexible ribs that gracefully moved out to the inside on the inhale, back expansion and everything. Textbook.

But I knew that was only one-third of the story. The next piece I wanted to understand was what her breathing mechanics were doing to her *Mix*, which in turn, would dictate the pH balance of her body, and therefore, give her headaches if left unchecked.

We hooked her up to my capnography biofeedback machine (that fancy device that measures the concentration of carbon dioxide in the exhalation). And there it was: Confirmed. Sara was breathing with beautiful mechanics... and using those same mechanics to over-breathe. I.e. hyperventilate.

By taking in a volume of air that was too high, she was blowing off too much CO_2, shifting her blood's acid-base balance, and, over time, that imbalance had crept off the mat and into her daily life. Her headache wasn't random, it was a chemistry problem she was unknowingly creating herself. And here's the wild part: she's not the only yogi I've seen do this. Sometimes, the very practice meant to center, focus and calm us end up subtly disrupting our entire system. Oops.

It was an easy fix. Before I tell you what it is, first, you need to understand the two unsung heroes in your body's breathing chemistry a little better: nitric oxide and carbon dioxide. Get to know them, and you're on the right track to respiring well. Let's roll.

Nitric Oxide: Your Built-In Performance Booster

Nitric oxide (NO) plays a massive role in breathing efficiency, cardiovascular health, and overall energy. It's produced primarily in your nasal passages, though your blood vessels make a bit of it too. But scientists didn't really grasp the scope of NO's importance until the late 1990s. That discovery was such a big deal that Murad, Furchgott, and Ignarro won the Nobel Prize in Physiology and Medicine in 1998 for uncovering its magic. [47-49]

I could stop here and just say: NO is your new best friend, and to get it, you need to breathe less, and you need to breathe through your nose. But let's go a little deeper.

NO is your body's behind-the-scenes fixer with a wide-reaching resume. In the cardiovascular system, NO is the reason your blood vessels stay relaxed and open. More NO, lower blood pressure, better heart function, and improved circulation. [50-52]

In the lungs, NO steps in again right where oxygen enters the bloodstream, to ease the transfer of oxygen from air to blood. It gets your oxygen exactly where it needs to go by helping your hemoglobin, the molecule that shuttles your oxygen around, do their job more efficiently.

But it doesn't stop there. Studies also show that NO helps fend off bacteria, viruses, and fungi, supports cellular repair, and acts as a potent antioxidant. We're talking immunity, recovery, and even longevity. [50-53]

You make it naturally by:

- Nose breathing: Every breath through your nose delivers nitric oxide straight into the lungs

- Regular exercise: Movement naturally signals your body to make more NO

- Eating your greens (and beets): Nitrate-rich veggies like beets, spinach, arugula, and kale are NO-building machines

- Humming: Research by Weitzberg, Lundberg and others have shown that humming can increase NO levels up to fifteen-fold. I've played around with fancy protocols, but here's what works best: hum a few minutes a day, a few times a day. [54-58]

Carbon Dioxide (CO_2) and Your Breathing Set Point

Alright, nitric oxide had its moment in the spotlight. Now let's shift the spotlight to a gas that's been seriously misunderstood: carbon dioxide. Our ideas about it are more than a little misguided. We've been doing CO_2 dirty.

First off, without it, you'd be dead. Quickly. Most people don't know this, but your urge to breathe doesn't primarily come from low oxygen, it comes from rising levels of CO_2. That's right. The thing we're always trying to get rid of is the very thing keeping us alive.

At the center of this life-saving process is a tiny, powerful structure in your brainstem called the pre-Bötzinger complex (and no, it's not a Bond villain). It's your breath's autopilot system. All day, every day, it monitors CO_2 levels in your blood, and when they rise? It sends the signal: "Okay, inhale now!" [59, 60]

No CO_2 signal, no breath. It's that simple.

But here's where it gets even more interesting: your brain's sensitivity to CO_2 is trainable. [61] Most people are overly sensitive to it, meaning even a tiny rise in CO_2 makes them feel like they need to take a big gulp of air. That's what leads to chronic over-breathing, which, as you now know, throws your body and mind into chaos.

With practice, you can learn to tolerate higher CO_2 levels. For example, free divers train their bodies to tolerate sky-high levels of CO_2 so they can hold their breath for five, sometimes even ten minutes. [62-64] (Not something to try without serious training!) Very impressive.

Your sensitivity to CO_2 is not set in stone. And adjusting it can unlock major improvements in your overall health.

But before we get to the fix, we need to understand one more key piece of the puzzle: The Bohr Effect, the chemistry behind how oxygen actually gets delivered where it's needed most.

How CO_2 Unlocks Your Oxygen (And Why That's a Big Deal)

Here's where breathing, chemistry, math, and physiology all collide in a way that can either make you feel incredible... or leave you foggy and fatigued.

Disclaimer: this story is about to get nerdy. In the early 1900s, two brilliant scientists named Christian Bohr and Lawrence Joseph Henderson were both working on the same puzzle: understanding how the body manages oxygen delivery.

Christian Bohr published his findings on what would become known as the Bohr Effect in 1904, showing that the more CO_2 present in the blood, the more easily hemoglobin releases oxygen. Around the same time (early 1900s through the 1910s), Lawrence Henderson was building what would become the Henderson–Hasselbalch equation, mathematically identifying the relationship between CO_2, bicarbonate, and blood pH. Essentially, Bohr identified what was happening, and Henderson mathematically explained how it was happening.

These two men never collaborated (being an ocean apart), but together they cracked the code for how your body handles oxygen delivery and pH regulation, stuff you feel every day whether you're sprinting, meditating, or lying in bed overthinking at 2 a.m.

The Bohr Effect shows that CO_2 and hydrogen ions (H^+) influence hemoglobin's ability to release oxygen into the tissues.

In simple terms, when CO_2 and H^+ levels are higher (like during exercise or focused mental work), hemoglobin loosens its grip on oxygen, allowing that oxygen to easily reach the cells. This is good. We need this to happen in order to stay healthy and perform well. When CO_2 levels are low, however, (like they are when you're over-breathing), the hemoglobin holds onto oxygen too tightly. Your blood might be full of oxygen, but it's locked up and unavailable to the tissues that need it most.

And how does that show up in real life? A few examples include brain fog, dizziness or lightheadedness, cold hands and feet (poor circulation), anxiety or a jitters, restless feelings, frequent sighing or yawning, tightness in the chest or feeling like you "can't get a full breath," and muscle fatigue that feels out of proportion to your effort. [3-7, 10, 65-69]

All signs that, despite plenty of oxygen in your system, your body can't use it efficiently. That's the Bohr Effect at work. That's your body waving a little red flag, asking you to stop breathing so much.

Want to test it out right now? Take five huge breaths, big in, big out. As big and full as you can.

That dizziness you feel is the result of the Bohr Effect. You have plenty of oxygen in your blood, but it's trapped. Your brain is literally starved for oxygen. Now breathe easily and let the dust settle. Your CO_2 will rise naturally, and hemoglobin will loosen its grip.

So, the next time you take a slow, small, and gentle breath and feel your body relax, and your state improve, you can silently toast Bohr, Henderson and his pal Hasselbalch... and whoever taught them chemistry.

How Shari Leveraged the Bohr Effect

Shari walked into my clinic looking frustrated and drained. As a medical billing specialist, she spent her days buried in codes, claims, and screens, but lately something felt off.

"I always catch myself not breathing," she admitted. "By lunchtime, I have headaches, and I feel exhausted. I think I need to learn how to breathe more."

It was a common assumption, one that had been drilled into her by "breathwork instructors" on social media. But as I ran some tests, the truth told a different story. Shari's Breath Fitness Score was 42 out of 100, far from ideal. And when we used a capnography biofeedback device to track her carbon dioxide levels, we saw the real culprit: Shari wasn't breathing too little, she was breathing too much. In short, her body was in a constant state of over-breathing, disrupting her chemistry and making her feel like she was running on fumes.

As I explained what was happening, something in Shari shifted. She went quiet, her eyes welling up with tears.

"So... it's not just in my head?" she whispered.

Not at all. The headaches, the exhaustion, the mental fog, it all made sense. The moment she realized this, it was like a massive weight had been lifted. Shari needed to breathe better and, surprisingly, that meant breathing less, especially when she was at rest.

With practice, she learned to comfortably slow down and soften her breath. Over time, her focus sharpened. Her energy levels stabilized. And those midday headaches that had plagued her for years?

"What headaches?" she said during our monthly check-in.

After working with Shari, I watched her go from someone constantly battling anxiety to someone who felt calm, grounded, and more in control. But this wasn't all sunshine and roses. Before we got to that stage, at the very beginning of her journey, she also said...

"David, I Feel Like Sh*t When I Try and Breathe Less"

I won't argue with this. Breathing less can feel downright awful at first, and when not done skillfully.

If CO_2 levels rise above your brain's comfort threshold, it sets off an intense panic response. Want proof? Just hold your breath well past that first urge to breathe. Within seconds, your body's alarm system kicks in. You may even get involuntary contractions in your belly. It's all very dramatic. But it's not because you're running out of oxygen. If we checked your blood's oxygen saturation, you'd likely still be sitting pretty (normal).

What's really happening? Your CO_2 levels are climbing, and your brain's breathing control center is not having it. To get you to breathe, it's flooding you with fear on purpose.

In 2013, researcher Oliver Feinstein and his team dropped a bombshell on our understanding of fear. They studied a woman known as S.M., who, due to a rare condition called Urbach-Wiethe disease, had completely lost both amygdalae (the brain's supposed fear centers). [70-72] Without them, S.M. was nearly fearless. Snakes, spiders, haunted houses... nothing fazed her.

But then they had her inhale air with 35% carbon dioxide (normal air has just 0.04%). Within seconds, she was having a panic attack. Her body's CO_2 sensors went haywire, proving that fear and panic can be triggered directly through rising CO_2 independent of the brain's traditional fear circuitry. Your body doesn't just think about danger; it feels it, chemically, without your consent. But why does this happen?

Back in the day for you as a caveperson, stress meant one thing: life-threatening danger. Usually physical. A big cat stalking you. An angry rival tribe. A flood, a fire, or something big and immediate. The body's response was simple: breathe faster, pump up adrenaline, and mobilize energy right now! No time to lose. This response readies the body for physical action (fight or flight).

Once the threat passed, everything settled down again. But fast forward to today... and we're not exactly dealing with these sorts of threats (most of the time). We're usually facing a different kind of predator: inboxes that never empty, bills that seem to breed on their own and the low hum of uncertainty in a world that never powers down.

These stressors aren't as intense as our primal problems were, but they're constant. Which is worse.

Guess what your body does to "help?" It breathes more. And more. And more. Just like it used to while running away from that hell panther, until the source of stress has disappeared. The kicker is that nowadays it doesn't leave. And we don't physically run it off or fight it out to help burn off the chemical soup. We just sit in it.

In short, over-breathing is your nervous system's way of surviving certain death. And it does this by hyperventilating.

So when we talk about learning to breathe less, let's start by cutting ourselves some slack. Our bodies are wired to keep us alive, and that means clinging to whatever coping strategies have worked, even if they're forty thousand years old and no longer helpful.

That's why we move forward with caution and compassion. No force. No breath-holding marathons. No heroic suffering.

We're here to retrain the system, to teach the brain, gently and consistently, that rising CO_2 isn't a threat.

How to Breathe Less Without Terrorizing Yourself

My friend and colleague, Robert Litman, founder of *The Breathable Body* [73], is brilliantly reluctant to tell people to "breathe less." In fact, he avoids it until people have demonstrated growing comfort and awareness of their breath. He fully understands the biochemistry behind breathing, and that of course people should breathe less, but he leans into the language we use around the practice.

I get it. The idea of "breathing less" can trip people up, making them tense or overthink the process. And if you've ever tried to breathe less by *trying* to breathe less, you probably know, it's not a good feeling and can make breath work feel like biological terrorism. I tend to be a bit more direct in my approach, but I carry Robert's voice and wisdom with me. His reminder: play nice with your breath.

To breathe less, we really only have two variables we can play with: breath rate (the speed of each breath) and breath volume (the amount of air you move with each breath).

The simplest formula? Breathe a little slower, a little lower in the body with a little less volume of air... and through your nose (that last part helps with the first three).

So go easy on yourself as you dive in now. And know that, just like Shari, you'll get it in the end!

Your Turn

Let's try this now.

Sit comfortably and upright. Let your tongue rest gently on the roof of your mouth. Breathe in and out through your nose.

Feel the inhale gently expand your lower ribs and lower abdomen.

And when you exhale, do it nice and slowly and smoothly.

Allow the movement of the lower ribs and lower belly to become just a little more subtle. Still there, still present, but without effort.

Settle into that rhythm and let it feel easy.

Try this for a couple of minutes before you read the next section.

You're Two Thirds In

You've got the full picture on breath Mechanics: how you breathe, as well as the biochemical Mix, what your body does once it's inside you. With those two pieces humming along, it's time to explore the final and perhaps most fascinating part of the breathing puzzle: the mind.

If Mechanics is the structure, and Mix is the chemical landscape, then Mind is the operator. It's the electrical system at the control panel, deciding how everything runs under pressure, in stillness, and everywhere in between.

It's the voice behind the breath, shaping how we respond to life moment by moment. Sometimes wisely, sometimes reactively. But when these three elements align? That's when the breath really starts to work for you.

I'll see you in the next chapter.

Activity 3: Qi Gong for CO_2 Tolerance

If you're serious about learning how to breathe less, and not in a "hold your breath and hope" kind of way, I've got something for you.

It's a short Qi Gong practice. Just a few minutes. But don't let the simplicity fool you. This practice is specifically designed to help regulate your breathing chemistry by calming your nervous system, reducing unnecessary muscular tension, and gently increasing your tolerance to carbon dioxide (without triggering panic or discomfort).

This particular sequence is designed to create space around your diaphragm, open your back and ribs, and coax your breath into a lower, slower, smoother rhythm without overthinking it.

You don't need special clothes. You don't need flexibility. You don't even need much time. Just a few minutes, an open mind, and the willingness to *do less* on purpose.

Go to breatheyourtruth.com/breathwork-exposed or scan the QR code below.

Chapter 4:
The Mind: The Psychophysiology of Breathing

EVER NOTICED HOW YOUR BREATH CHANGES with your mood?

Nervous? It's shallow and sharp. Calm? It's slow and smooth. That's no accident. Your breath and your mind are in constant conversation. The mind races, and the breath speeds ups (or reacts). But the breath also *talks back* to the mind. Slow the breath and it calms the mind, speed up the breath and it excites the mind. Change one, you influence the other.

This is why ancient traditions like Qi Gong, Yoga, and meditation have always leaned on breathwork to settle or simulate the mind. And why modern research is finally catching up, showing how subtle breath shifts can rewire stress patterns, steady emotions, and sharpen focus.

So, in this chapter, we'll explore the third and final M. It's the cherry on top of your breathing Mechanics and Mix, the piece that ties it all together.

Let's start by understanding the first link between the breath and the mind.

Link 1: Your Autonomic Nervous System

The ANS plays a crucial role in how we feel both physically and emotionally. It governs which organ systems are activated and which are relaxed. It's like the operating system running quietly in the background, regulating everything from your heartbeat to digestion, all without needing your conscious input. It's the part of you that holds the show together while you're busy doing... anything else.

Even though it's called "autonomic" (as if it runs *automatically*) it's fascinating to realize that key parts are under our control, if we're bold enough to take the reins.

To keep things digestible, let's break the ANS into two major branches. (There's more nuance here, *looking at you, polyvagal theory*, but for now, let's say there are two.)

The first is the Sympathetic Nervous System (SNS): your "get up and go" or "get to the party" system. It kicks in when you're excited, needing to focus, anxious, in danger, or just running late for a meeting. It speeds things up, heart rate, breath rate, alertness, all in the name of rallying the troops for bigger living, or survival.

On the other side of the coin is the Parasympathetic Nervous System (PNS): this is your "rest and digest" system. It slows some things down while waking other parts up. It signals safety, aids digestion, and supports healing. In short, it tells your body, "Hey, you're okay now. Time to breathe easy."

Most systems in your body respond automatically to the ANS, but your breath can relay information back to it. And the vagus nerve is your direct line.

The vagus nerve is a wandering cranial nerve that is the major highway connecting your breath to your brain, organs, and emotional system. It responds especially well to slow, deep, diaphragmatic breathing. We'll get into what that looks and feels like soon. But for now, remember this: your breath is like a remote control of your nervous system. Most people don't even know it's there, but once you realize you've got it, with practice, you can change the channel anytime, waking things up or calming things down.

Link 2: Your Nose

It's wild how often we overlook it, but your nose is basically your body's built-in tranquility switch. The gatekeeper of your "rest and digest" mode (the parasympathetic nervous system), if you will. Sure, it filters, humidifies, and warms the air, but you're about to see how that only scratches the surface.

When you breathe through your nose, you're dialing into the activation of the parasympathetic nervous system and in the right context, quieting your "fight or flight" setting. That is thanks, in part, to how nasal breathing adds helpful resistance to the incoming airflow. This nudges your diaphragm into action, helping you breathe lower and slower. That also generally means more CO_2 and therefore, better chemistry.

Lastly, there are neural connections from the nasal passages to the brain that help regulate our nervous system. [28, 30, 74, 75] That's a triple-win for nervous system balance. In fact, it's hard to nose-breathe in a way that's gentle and rhymical and be freaking out in a whirlwind of anxiety at the same time. The wiring just doesn't work that way.

Breathing through the nose has been a core part of Yoga, Qi Gong, and meditation practices for centuries, even though the science has been a bit slower to catch up.

Take alternate nostril breathing (called *nadi shodhana* in Yoga). It has been shown to improve heart rate variability (HRV), a strong marker of nervous system resilience and general health. [51, 76, 77] When HRV goes up, your body's ability to adapt and recover improves. Think: more calm, less overwhelm, pretty quickly.

Let's give it a go right now.

Take a moment and switch to breathing only through your nose. Don't try to change anything else for now. Just notice what happens.

Can you feel things slow down a notch? Does the breath feel quieter? Maybe your jaw releases, or your shoulders drop just a little.

That's your nervous system responding.

Let's go deeper and try alternate nostril breathing:

- Gently block your right nostril with your right thumb, and inhale through the left nostril only. Breathe in until you feel your belly has expanded, but don't force it
- Now block the left nostril with your right ring finger and release your thumb from your right nostril
- Exhale through the right nostril only, until your lungs feel mostly empty
- Inhale through the right nostril again, then block it with your thumb
- Unblock the left by removing your ring finger and exhale through the left side
- Inhale through the left nostril, and at the top of the inhale, switch nostrils

Repeat this a few times. If in doubt, just remember to switch nostrils after you have taken your inhale. And don't take huge, long, breaths. You don't have to fill your lungs here. Let the breath stay soft and subtle. Let it feel good. Let it feel easy. And notice what happens.

Link 3: Your Diaphragm

If you enjoyed that, you'll love what's coming next.

When it comes to regulating the nervous system, few muscles matter more than your diaphragm. But as you well know, most people aren't using it fully. Life tends to stack tension in the shoulders, lock the ribs, and pull breath up into the chest. By overriding the diaphragm, it ends up stiff and underused.

When the diaphragm is active, I mean fully moving, it does more than just pull air into your lungs. Because the vagus nerve runs through the diaphragm, when it moves, it sends a powerful message up to the brain that says you're safe and there's no need to be stressed. Some systems quiet down, like the heart and the big muscles of the body, while others finally get a chance to shine, like peripheral vision, digestion, even sexual function.

And here's the coolest part of using your diaphragm correctly: it moves your *brain*. Literally. When your diaphragm engages, it creates a pressure shift that reaches down into your abdomen and all the way up your spine. That pressure travels through the spinal canal, nudging the cerebrospinal fluid upwards (the clear liquid that cushions and nourishes your brain). That movement is a good thing. It supports your brain health by improving circulation and clearing waste. [30] Use your diaphragm well, and it becomes tonic for your nervous system and a massage for your brain.

In Traditional Chinese Medicine and Qi Gong, the diaphragm region is considered a key energy hub, one that promotes your mental wellbeing. Now you can see why. [78]

The more you practice using your diaphragm, the more it shows up when you need it most: during stress, activity, or emotional overwhelm. It becomes a stabilizing anchor, not just for your breath, but for your whole experience of life.

When nasal and diaphragmatic breathing are paired together, they create a powerful synergy that enhances your overall health more effectively than either practice alone. For many, this pairing has been truly medicinal as they sought to overcome the most debilitating mental health conditions, including the most prevalent one of our time: anxiety.

How James Found His Antidote to Anxiety

James worked in tech support for a public utility company. He was sharp, kind, and carried the wear-and-tear of long days troubleshooting everyone else's problems. His wife was the one who nudged him my way.

"He seems out of breath," she said, "even when he's just sitting."

James described it plainly: "It gets worse as the work-week goes on. By Friday, it feels like I'm suffocating. I'm not sure what a panic attack is, but I think I've had a few."

Now, I'm a physical therapist, not a mental health professional. But I also know that unaddressed anxiety often shows up as breathing dysfunction, and *that's* squarely in my wheelhouse. Within minutes, I could see James's breath frequently moved high in his chest. Especially when he took a breath right before speaking.

He didn't have a reliable sense of when he was mouth breathing either. His resting CO_2 levels were low. And when we ran a hyperventilation test, just ten big breaths, his system fell apart. His recovery was painfully slow to get back to his baseline.

This told me two things: One, his autonomic nervous system was already on edge, and two, his body had lost its ability to recover from even minor disruptions quickly.

The good news? We had two clear targets: Mechanics (how he was breathing) and Mix (his chemistry). We agreed he'd track the Mind part as we worked together to change his breathing patterns.

We started small. James focused on building tolerance to nose breathing during low-effort tasks like replying to emails and practiced gentle breath awareness while walking. He didn't feel a dramatic shift right away, but within two weeks, his data told a quieter truth. His resting CO_2 levels improved and his tolerance to nose breathing increased, among other positive side effects.

"I think I'm sleeping better," he told me one day, rubbing his neck like he didn't quite believe it. "But I still crash by the end of the week. It's like my system hasn't caught up yet."

It was true. On the outside, things were starting to change. But on the inside, his nervous system was still learning it was safe to breathe correctly. Then, around week eight, something clicked.

"I think I've got this," he said. At times, he could still feel the familiar tightening his chest and general sense of unease but now, that was becoming a trigger for steady breathing. The breath that once spiraled into panic had steadied and his nervous system (once in a near-constant state of surveillance) had started to recalibrate. And most importantly, he stopped treating his body like the enemy. He started trusting it again.

We kept going. Once James had dialed in his nose breathing, lower-body mechanics, and improved his CO_2 levels, his Breath Fitness Score climbed from forty to fifty-six in just a few weeks. That was our green light to up our game. Time to introduce resonant breathing.

Enter, Resonant Breathing

This is where things got interesting.

Resonant breathing is a gentle practice of breathing at a pace that helps the heart, lungs, and nervous system fall into rhythm. This would help reduce James' anxiety even further.

Resonant breathing involved training James' body to only take around six breaths per minute (as opposed to the seventeen or more he was inhaling before). Most people today breathe twelve to twenty times per minute. [79] That's way too much. I told him that resonant breathing looked like breathing in for around five seconds and exhaling for another five seconds. That would equate to approximately six breaths per minute. Simple. But at first, it was rocky for James.

He couldn't sustain six breaths per minute for more than two minutes without me watching his CO_2 levels crash. Not good. Yes, he slowed his breathing down, but he took in more air with each breath, unintentionally hyperventilating. I knew it wouldn't serve him. So, we adjusted. Shorter sessions, just two minutes at a time, a few times a day. Just enough to nudge his system gently forward. The cue I gave him?

"Let it feel like underachieving."

He played with that idea for a week. Then, a shift. A week later, James could sustain five full minutes of resonant breathing without his CO_2 levels dropping. His nervous system was learning to stay steady in the face of change, and his anxiety was reducing.

How did resonant breathing help him? It all came down to rhythm. When you breathe at a slower pace, anywhere around 4.5

to 7.5 breaths per minute, in a gentle, rhymical way, something powerful happens in your body. Your heart rate begins to gently speed up when you inhale and slow down when you exhale. That natural rise and fall is called heart rate variability (HRV), and it's a key sign of a healthy, balanced nervous system.

Think of it like a Waltz between your breath and your heart. The smoother the dance, the more adaptable and resilient your body becomes to stress of any kind. Resonant breathing is the tempo that brings it all into harmony. [80]

When practiced regularly with good breath mechanics and healthy CO_2 levels, resonant breathing becomes a powerful reset button for your entire system. It lowers blood pressure and heart rate, improves heart rate variability and baroreceptor sensitivity, and stimulates the vagus nerve. The effects ripple outward: less anxiety, more emotional resilience, and a general sense of steadiness in both body and mind.

Check out the instructions I gave to James, and try it yourself:

- First, let your breath become softer, steadier, and lower like a quiet ripple beneath the surface
- Inhale gently through your nose for four to five seconds, feeling your diaphragm area and lower ribs expand
- Exhale just as softly, through your nose, for five to six seconds. No pushing. No forcing. Keep it low in the body. And keep the volume light

That's it. That's how you honor the mechanics and the mix and unlock the deeper potential of your breath, and its mastery over your mind.

If you've been paying very close attention, you might be getting a little suspicious right about now. *Wait a second...* you're thinking. If subtle, slow, rhythmic breathing builds resilience and raises CO_2 tolerance, then what about all those big, fast, buzzy breathwork techniques that are blowing up on social media?

You know the ones. The ones with ice baths, booming soundtracks, and people breathing like steam engines before declaring their third eye just opened.

Aren't those doing the opposite of everything we've just covered? you ask.

Well, yes, in a way. That's exactly where we're headed in quite a bit of depth in the next chapter.

But in the same vein as resonant breathing, there's one more breathing exercise that is excellent for the mind that's worth mentioning in this chapter.

Another Breathwork Technique That's Worth the Hype (When Done Properly)

Sometimes called "square breathing," box breathing is one of the most widely used breath control techniques in the world. It shows up in Yoga studios, athletic training rooms, and even military operations. Former Navy SEAL Commander Mark Divine helped bring it into the spotlight, using it to help soldiers stay calm and focused under pressure. [81] If it works for those in combat, there's a good chance it'll help you manage your stressful day at work.

The practice itself is simple: Inhale for four seconds. Hold for four. Exhale for four. Hold again for four. Then repeat.

If that's too easy, try five, six or seven seconds.

That's it. The even timing and consistent pacing give your overactive brain something to focus on. It anchors your attention and dials down mental noise. But real magic happens under the hood.

Box breathing slows your breathing rate, which usually means you retain more CO_2. That's a good thing as you know. I regularly see my clients improve their CO_2 tolerance, recover better and gain greater nervous system flexibility if they stick with it and practice properly.

BUT and this is a really big but... you will get the best results IF you are inhaling *gently*, with a *small* volume of air. Because slower isn't always better if each breath is too big.

Another point worth mentioning is that box breathing isn't how you should breathe all day either. It's not your background breath while walking the dog or making coffee. It's a tool, not a template. It should be a short, focused activity no longer than fifteen minutes per day. Just like you wouldn't spend all day in the gym, you wouldn't spend all day doing this!

Box breathing isn't perfect. No breathwork methodology is. But for most people, this one offers low risk and high reward for your body and your mind when compared to the rest.

So far, we've been predominantly exploring how the breath can make or break your mind, and what we should be avoiding in order to protect ourselves. But we're missing an angle.

The Breath Affects the Mind, and the Mind Affects the Breath

Now that we've explored how the breath can influence the mind, it's time to turn the mirror around. Because just as the breath shapes our mental state, our thoughts, emotions, and inner stories shape the way we breathe.

Before we dive in, I want to offer a quick note of context. I'm trained as a physical therapist, not a psychologist or licensed mental health professional. I don't diagnose mental health conditions, and I don't claim to have answers when it comes to the complex terrain of the mind. But what I do have is over a few decades of experience working with real people, in real stress states, and watching, again and again, how mental health shows up in the body and breath.

Ever notice how your breath behaves when you're anxious or self-critical? It gets tight, short, up in the chest. When you're rushing, worrying, or overthinking, your breath tends to reflect that state, becoming fragmented, shallow, or even erratic. The body responds as if it's under threat, even when the "danger" is just an unfinished to-do list or an awkward conversation on the horizon.

On the flip side, when we feel calm, safe, and present, the breath naturally slows. It drops lower in the body. It becomes quieter, more rhythmic. This is the feedback loop we live in every day. Your emotions listen to your breath. But your breath is also listening to your emotions. So, the question becomes: how can we gently influence the breath, not just through overt breath mechanics, but by bringing awareness to our minds and our emotions?

First off, it's helpful to see the breath as a reflection; a moment-to-moment messenger of what's happening inside us. It tells the truth, whether we like that truth or not. And that makes it one of the most honest, and humble teachers we have.

Sometimes that truth is inconvenient. You sit down to meditate and discover a restless mind and a choppy breath. You go for a walk, thinking you're fine, and suddenly realize you're mouth breathing and worrying about something. The breath doesn't flatter the ego. It shows us what's actually going on.

Try it yourself by pausing. Feel your breath. Don't control it. Don't perform. Just meet it. Notice where it lives in your body. Is it high, low, or centered? Fast or slow? Tight or soft? Then take it one step further. Ask, "What is this breath telling me about how I'm feeling?"

Don't worry if the answer isn't clear. Just hold the question and let the observation do its quiet work.

This simple act, observing your breath and staying open to its message, is gold, even if you discover an inconvenient truth. Remember, this state isn't permanent. It's just how things are *right now*. And noticing it? That's where change begins.

As you continue to observe your breath, you may notice your mind at work. Perhaps it fixates on one subject, flits between many, or sometimes focuses beautifully. Whatever its tendency, simply observe it. Each time you realize your mind has wandered, gently reorient your focus back to your breath and notice it intertwined with your mind. In doing so, you create space for your mind to transform your breath.

Can you feel any difference?

That's meditation. It's fundamentally a practice of self-honesty. This kind of breath awareness is deceptively simple but over time, it builds a new connection between you and your breath. You stop seeing the breath as a performance and start seeing it as a companion.

Let's try something else for fun. This is one of my favorite real-life breathwork practices. It's not just about breathing well, it's about syncing your breath with the emotion you *want* to feel, or with the "story" you want to embody. Here's how to try it:

Step 1: Breathe Well

- First, check in with your breath
- Breathe in and out through your nose
- Let the breath stay low in the body. Aim for the lower ribs, solar plexus, or belly
- Go slightly slower than your normal pace. Just a little
- Keep it soft and quiet. No forcing or straining
- If you feel the need for a big deep breath now and then? That's fine. Let it reset you

Step 2: Choose Your Story

Now choose a feeling, mindset, or inner narrative that you want to carry into your day. This doesn't have to be a literal story. It could be a simple emotional tone or intention, like:

- "Life wants everything to be great for me"
- "I'm calm and capable"
- "I'm full of happiness and gratitude"

- "I'm compassionate and loving toward myself"
- "I'm safe, even when things are hard"
- "I'm grounded; the ground is here for me"

It can be a word, a sentence, or even just a feeling you imagine spreading through your chest. No need to overthink it. Pick something that feels needed.

Step 3: Pair Your Breath with That Story

Now, gently bring the two together. As you breathe, imagine your chosen story, or the emotion you want to feel, flowing in with each inhale and anchoring deeper into your body with each exhale. Let it ride the rhythm of your breath, like a quiet current.

Ask yourself: If I truly believed this story, how would my body be breathing right now? Would it be slower? Softer? Longer? Let your breath reflect that without pushing or performing.

The aim isn't to fake a feeling, but to allow your breath and your story to gradually align.

Then, try sprinkling this throughout your day. In real life. In motion. Try it:

- While waiting for a webpage to load
- As you get in or out of your car
- In line at the café or grocery store
- As you pause before answering a message

These micro-moments are perfect training grounds. You don't need to stop what you're doing. Just return to your breath, recall your story, and let them meet quietly in the background.

It's true that many of us must swim upstream from our own biology. We're hardwired for negativity. Nature made it more important to stay safe than to stay happy. The awesome part? You're free to outsmart your biology if you'd like.

One day, you may catch yourself walking into a tough conversation or stressful moment, and instead of tightening up, your breath will stay calm because you think of your story and your breath will follow you.

Activity 4: Bringing the Triple M Together

Now you've made it through the Triple M Triangle, it's time to turn it up a notch and bring those lessons off the page and into your body.

Enter Qi Gong. At its core, Qi Gong is a practice that integrates all three M's in real time. Through gentle, natural movement, conscious breath, and relaxed attention, you begin to embody everything you've learned. Your mechanics sharpen. Your chemistry steadies. Your mind settles. This is why Qi Gong has become my go-to reset. I use it between breath coaching sessions, before writing, or at the end of the day when I need to come back to center.

I've created a short, accessible Qi Gong sequence that brings the Triple M Triangle to life. Go to breatheyourtruth.com/breathwork-exposed, or scan the QR code below, look for Activity 4, and join me for a few quiet minutes.

Chapter 5:
Where Breathwork Magic Meets Breathwork Misinformation

NOW WE'RE READY TO STEP INTO the more intense, dramatic corner of the breathwork world. It's time to address the elephant in the room.

If what we've learned so far is that most of us are over breathing, and that's negatively affecting our mental and physical health... what are these breathwork teachers doing making us over breathe on purpose? Whether it's for stress relief, spiritual awakening, or peak performance, modern breathwork's solution is often the same: *Breathe more, breathe harder.*

Many breathwork instructors have one tool in their belt and call it a toolbox. One technique, one narrative, and often, one weekend certification. No shame, many mean well, but most haven't been taught how to assess breath fitness, let alone build it.

If you've tried one of these bold breathwork practices and walked away underwhelmed or over-wired you're not alone. Plenty of these techniques work... until they don't. Especially when used out of context, on the wrong foundation, or by someone who hasn't done their own breathing homework on these methods and assessed their clinical results on the majority.

You've probably heard of them. The Wim Hof Method, known for its icy grit and powerful breath holds. Rebirthing, designed to "heal trauma" and promote deep emotional release. Then there are ancient techniques from Yoga and Buddhist philosophies, developed to induce spiritual enlightenment. The list goes on. What ties these styles together is their intentional use of big, fast, and forceful breathing usually through the mouth, well beyond your body's metabolic needs. It's conscious over-breathing, and it's designed to shake things up.

There's some research showing breathwork like this can temporarily sharpen alertness and give you a kind of neurological "reset." That's real, and for the *right* person, it can be a good thing.

But here's the part that rarely gets talked about: they come with major trade-offs. Especially if your baseline breath is still in recovery. (Most of us sit in this camp.) For one, these practices *intentionally* lower your CO_2, which isn't what we want in general, is it?

They can also make the pH of your blood rise to unhealthy levels. Not ideal.

They can deeply disrupt your heart rate variability (HRV) as well. Bad news for anxiety-sufferers.

Plus, they can easily, over time, override your natural breathing rhythm and nervous system regulation (which can make skilled, subtle breathing harder to access post-breathwork).

Therefore, while hyperventilation breathwork can be useful for our mental health in short bursts... is it worth the long-term consequences, the dangers, for most *normal* people? Probably not.

Take my client James as an example. When he first walked into my clinic, his breathing was already dysregulated. He was over-breathing by default, had low CO_2 tolerance, and his nervous system was stuck in a subtle, chronic stress and anxiety loop. If I had given him one of these breathwork practices at that point, say The Wim Hof Method, it would've been like throwing gasoline on a flame. For James, it wouldn't have only been completely useless, but borderline dangerous for his health.

That doesn't mean these practices are "bad," just that they're not for everyone, perhaps even most people, especially not in the beginning stages of breath retraining.

This chapter is your decoder ring. Not a takedown, but a translation. Because ultimately and ideally, we want practices that go further than just distracting our nervous systems. It's also about finding a long-term solution for what you're hoping these breathwork modalities will heal in you. We'll explore the major breathwork categories, how they impact your body and brain, what risks they carry, and what kind of preparation helps them work better (or at all). Welcome to your breathwork magic and misinformation map.

The Four Breathwork Categories

Before we explore specific breath practices, let's get our bearings.

Breathwork isn't one thing. It's a wide, messy landscape filled with techniques that pull different strings in the body. Some settle the mind. Some spike your nervous system. Some mess with your blood chemistry. Others tune up your core strength. To help you make sense of it, I've found it useful to break breathwork into four primary categories, each one targeting a different main focus or purpose.

Categorizing and understanding these practices gives you more control over your own experience, like adjusting the dials on a soundboard. Each breathwork technique targets different aspects of health and performance, but the controls are all connected. Turn one knob, and you'll influence the others, amplifying, softening, or shifting the entire mix. We'll start off on a positive, shall we? Here are the four categories of breathwork and what's great about them.

Category	Primary Focus	How It's Done	What It's Great For
Mindful Breathing	Awareness	Observing breath, body, emotions and thoughts	Reducing stress, improving focus, emotional regulation
Respiratory Strength Muscle Training	Biomechanics	Strengthening breathing muscles and spine support	Boosting endurance, posture, and mechanical efficiency
Under-Breathing (Breathing Less)	Biochemistry	Reducing the breath, building tolerance to CO_2, efficiency and conservation	Fixing chronic over breathing, shortness of breath, anxiety, digestive problems, breaking performance plateaus
Over-Breathing (Hyper-ventilation)	Psycho-physiology	Big, fast, or cyclical continuous breathing exceeding the metabolic need	Altering mental states, accessing emotions, releasing tension

Let's take a closer look at each one, starting with one of the quiet heavyweights in the breathwork world.

Mindful Breathing

Mindfulness is the practice of paying attention on purpose, in the present moment, and without judgment. It's not about clearing your mind (which is a near-on impossible feat anyway!). It's about noticing what's actually happening: sensations, thoughts, and feelings as they arise, without immediately trying to fix, fight, or flee.

Paying attention to the breath is the most common anchor to the sitting version of this practice. Remember, your breath is a mirror. When you're tense, it gets tight. When you're calm, it softens. By watching the breath, you're watching the nervous system in action. And by staying present with it without trying to control it, you're strengthening your ability to stay steady and aware, even when things get uncomfortable.

At first glance, mindfulness breathing seems simple: Just sit, notice your breath coming in and out, and stay present. If you drift, come back. Done. But it's an advanced practice in disguise.

Why? Because simply observing your breath without changing it is way harder than it sounds. We're wired to do, fix, and manage. Just being with the breath without judgment is a skill. And like most skills worth having, it takes practice.

You'll probably catch yourself tweaking the breath the moment you notice it. Or judging it as too shallow, too fast, too something. Or drifting off to mentally rehash that awkward conversation or remember what you forgot at the grocery store. It's totally normal to spend twenty minutes "being mindful" and realize you were present for two of them. I've been there. Often. Another thing that shows up is a sense of breath claustrophobia. You're not quite sure if you should breathe more or less to feel better. That, too, is part of the process and workable. Over time, this gets easier, and the benefits start flooding in.

This style of breathwork forms the backbone of the Mindfulness-Based Stress Reduction (MBSR) program, created in 1979 by Jon Kabat-Zinn at the University of Massachusetts Medical Center. It's one of the most well-researched and effective mind-body practices for reducing stress, anxiety, and improving general well-being. [82]

Respiratory Muscle Strength Training (RMST)

On the surface, Respiratory Muscle Strength Training (RMST) looks a lot like strength training for your breath, and that's exactly what it is. Just like you would train your legs to run faster or your arms to lift heavier, RMST focuses on strengthening the muscles that power your inhale and exhale, stabilize your spine, and support your posture.

RMST was originally developed to help people with chronic respiratory diseases like COPD and asthma. [83] Over time, though, it caught the attention of athletes and trainers for a simple reason: stronger, better-coordinated breathing muscles mean better endurance, improved posture, and less fatigue across the board. Whether you're climbing a flight of stairs or sprinting toward a finish line, breathing strength matters. And it's trainable.

There are two main ways RMST challenges the system. The first is an indirect challenge by adding resistance to airflow itself. Think of breathing through something that makes inhaling and exhaling harder, forcing your muscles to work overtime. The second is a direct challenge by adding resistance directly to the breathing muscles through specific postures, efforts, or external devices. Both approaches aim to build control, efficiency, and resilience under pressure.

There's now a growing range of tools designed to make this kind of training possible. Devices like the SportsMask from The Oxygen Advantage®, the Airofit breathing trainer, the Breather Fit, or spirometers provide indirect resistance, making you work harder to move the same amount of air. Others, like the Buteyko Belt or simple training postures (even breathing while holding a handstand!) create direct load on the muscles themselves, strengthening the diaphragm, intercostals, and supporting musculature like the chest, back, and neck.

A quick word of caution: many of the popular RMST devices encourage mouth breathing. You know how I feel about mouth breathing. That might be fine for short, targeted training sessions for super-breathers, but I always encourage nasal breathing whenever possible to preserve good breathing habits and chemistry in the long run.

When applied wisely, RMST offers some impressive benefits. Over time, it can significantly improve your breathing muscle efficiency, making breathing feel easier and more sustainable during both exercise and rest. It also supports better spinal stability and posture, because yes, your breathing muscles are deeply connected to your core strength. And perhaps most importantly, it enhances respiratory endurance, making you more resilient whether you're rehabilitating from an illness, training for performance, or just trying to navigate daily life with more energy and ease. [83]

Strengthening your breathing muscles might not sound flashy. But it's one of the smartest, most sustainable investments you can make in your health, your movement, and your longevity.

Under-Breathing or Breathing Less

To the untrained ear (and nose) the idea of *under-breathing* sounds like something to avoid. But as you well know, most people today aren't breathing too little. They're breathing too *much,* too fast, too shallow, and too often, shooting themselves in the foot and disrupting their body's chemical balance. Under-breathing practices aim to restore that balance.

By breathing slightly less than you're used to (closer to what your body actually needs) you create the chemical conditions that encourage oxygen to be released from hemoglobin and delivered where it's needed most.

Under-breathing also builds biochemical resilience: The ability to stay calm, clear, and in control even when your body starts sending desperate signals for more air. It's training your chemistry to work *for* you, not against you.

Some of the key elements of strategically breathing less include:

- Reduced breathing volume or rate: Slow, light, quiet nasal breathing that matches your true metabolic needs, not your mind's anxiety-driven demands. It also includes exaggerated reduced breathing volume and rate to intentionally stress the body.

- Controlled breath holds: Gentle pauses after an exhale to help raise CO_2 levels safely and retrain your tolerance for chemical discomfort. It also includes more aggressive breath holding – done with safety guidelines.

- Nasal breathing focus: Almost always through the nose. This maintains natural filtration, keeps nitric oxide production strong, and protects your breathing mechanics.

- A calm mental state: Under-breathing practices prioritize staying calm and recovering smoothly – for light, and aggressive practices.

- Silent mechanics: No dramatic chest pumping or belly thrusts. Just soft, low movement felt deep in the ribs, abdomen, and back

Here are a few standout examples.

The Buteyko Method

This is the heavyweight of the "breathe less" movement. Originally developed by Soviet physician Dr. Konstantin Buteyko in the 1950s to treat asthma and respiratory conditions, it focuses on nasal breathing, slowing your breath, and building CO_2 tolerance as a fundamental marker of health. [11, 84, 85]

For most people, mastering the Buteyko method can be transformational, with deep, powerful shifts in chemistry, energy, and resilience. That said, sometimes the method is taught a little rigidly, focusing purely on the numbers and missing the emotional, somatic experience of breathing. In my experience, when it's paired with a broader, embodied understanding of the breath, the core Buteyko principles become an essential pillar of real Breath Fitness.

How do you practice it?

- You breathe through your nose at all times: day and night, including during exercise

- You slow your breath until it becomes light, quiet, and almost invisible
- You practice "control pauses" (small, gentle breath holds after a normal exhale to gradually raise your CO_2 tolerance and retrain your brain and body to feel safe with less air)
- You stay calm and relaxed the whole time. No straining. No pushing. No turning blue

Let me break down that "control pause":

- Breathe normally through your nose for a few breaths
- After a normal (not forced) exhale, gently hold your breath
- Time how many seconds it takes before you feel the first natural urge to breathe (not when you're gasping, just the first clear signal)
- Then, resume calm, soft nasal breathing

Over time, the goal is to increase the duration of that control pause. This will build your CO_2 tolerance and stabilize your breathing patterns in daily life, not just during practice, but all the time.

Done properly, Buteyko work opens the door to deeper, more efficient oxygenation by *untraining* the chronic over-breathing that modern life wires into us.

Intermittent Hypoxia Training (IHT)

At first glance, Intermittent Hypoxia Training (IHT) sounds intimidating, and truthfully, it can be. It's deliberate, controlled exposure to short periods of lower oxygen and elevated CO_2. Think of it like biochemical weightlifting for your breath: brief stress, followed by recovery, designed to build real resilience at a chemical and cellular level. IHT can rapidly improve CO_2 tolerance, boost oxygen efficiency, spike erythropoietin (EPO) production (which helps your body make more red blood cells), and strengthen your breathing muscles all without damaging your baseline breathing patterns. [61, 86-88]

Other potential benefits include better sprint performance, stronger diaphragmatic function, more efficient energy production, and even possible therapeutic effects for conditions like sleep apnea and certain forms of fatigue. [61, 86, 88-97]

That said, IHT isn't risk-free. Done incorrectly or too aggressively, it can cause oxidative stress, strain the cardiovascular system, or worsen anxiety. That's why I recommend reaching a Breath Fitness Score of at least seventy before incorporating this type of training. You want a good baseline of breathing resilience before you start layering stressful practices.

How do you practice IHT? The simplest way is to play with small breath holds:

- Start with light nasal breathing to settle your system
- After a normal exhale (not forced), gently hold your breath
- Time how many seconds you can comfortably hold (you're looking for a manageable urge to breathe, not full-blown stomach contractions and gasping)
- When you feel that first strong but controlled urge, resume calm, quiet nasal breathing
- Rest and recover fully between holds (at least one or two minutes of easy breathing)
- Repeat for 3–5 rounds
- Set the intention to expand your hold time (over time)

In a more advanced IHT practice, you might pair breath holds with light to moderate movement, like walking, squatting, or jogging. This adds another layer of demand and can create even bigger gains in breathing efficiency and CO_2 tolerance, but only when your system is ready for it.

The key is gradual exposure. IHT should feel like a challenge, not a whirlwind of panic.

Oxygen Advantage®

Patrick McKeown's *Oxygen Advantage* program is a brilliant evolution of the Buteyko Method and Intermittent Hypoxic Training (IHT). Patrick took rigorous breathing science (once the domain of clinicians and elite performance labs) and made it usable for athletes, coaches, and everyday people who just want to perform better and feel better. [13, 98]

Oxygen Advantage is about training your body to become more efficient with less air. It focuses heavily on using breath holds strategically, especially during exercise, to simulate the effects of high-altitude training. This controlled stress triggers the body to adapt, producing more red blood cells, improving oxygen efficiency, and enhancing both aerobic and anaerobic endurance. His sprint-hold protocol, in particular, has been shown to improve repeated-sprint performance in as little as two weeks.

It's smart, scalable, and supported by research. It's also incredibly practical; there's no need for fancy equipment, no extreme sessions, just deliberate, intelligent training. I'm happy to report that I've personally contributed to Oxygen Advantage over the years, and I include Patrick's approach in my collection of training.

Here's the basic structure of a classic *Oxygen Advantage* sprint-hold session:

- Warm up gently. Walk or jog lightly for a few minutes to get your system moving
- After a normal exhale, hold your breath. Not a deep, forced exhale, just a regular, comfortable one
- Once you exhale, pinch your nose and hold your breath while you walk or jog slowly
- Continue holding your breath until you feel air hunger. You're aiming for a moderate to strong urge to breathe
- Release the hold and breathe in through your nose once you feel you really need to
- Recover fully with easy, nasal breathing. Give yourself at least 30–60 seconds, or longer if needed, until your breathing feels settled again
- Repeat for up to 10 rounds

Over time, as your CO_2 tolerance improves, you'll be able to hold your breath longer and recover faster.

There are a few important guidelines to keep in mind as you practice. Always prioritize quality recovery between holds; the recovery phase is just as important as the hold itself. Never force the session. If your body is signaling that it needs to stop, listen. Stay nasal throughout, both during the active phases and the recovery periods, to support proper mechanics and chemistry.

Freediving

Freediving breath training isn't just about holding your breath for long periods; it's about mastering calm under real pressure. It's a mental discipline that demands presence, patience, and a deep respect of your own physiology.

Modern freediving is both a sport and an art form. But historically, it was about survival. Ancient cultures dove under the sea for food, sometimes pearls, sponges, and even for strategic military operations. Plato and Homer mentioned freedivers in ancient Greece. The Japanese Ama divers, mostly women, have been harvesting from the sea for over two thousand years without tanks or gear. [99]

And here's the critical point: the most successful freedivers survived by breathing less and breathing better. Pre-dive hyperventilation (huge inhales before a dive) is actually dangerous. It drops CO_2 levels too much, dulls your natural warning signals, and can lead to shallow water blackout. Freediving teaches you the opposite: build resilience to rising CO_2, learn to stay calm in discomfort, and respect the moment your body tells you, "It's time to breathe."

The essence of freediving training isn't complicated, but it requires discipline and respect for your body's signals.

To start, you just breathe normally before you submerge yourself under the water, calming your system rather than overloading it. No deep breaths or hyperventilation whatsoever. You breathe out fully, then, once underwater, it's about staying calm and listening closely to the subtle cues your body gives you, surfacing well before you reach your absolute limit.

The benefits of freediving go way beyond just holding your breath for a party trick. You build serious CO_2 tolerance and you train your nervous system to stay calm under highs stakes, even when the past version of you would have hit the panic button. Plus, there's something magical about slipping underwater, unplugging from the noise of life, and realizing you can be so much more resilient than you thought.

All that being said, do NOT try this without a trained professional guiding you in a series of legit classes. This is not something to just "experiment" with on your own.

Over-Breathing (Hyperventilation)

Now, the section you've been waiting for. Of all the categories of breathwork, none is more practiced, more misunderstood, or more abused than intentional over-breathing.

It's dramatic. It's intense. And it often comes with a euphoric punch at the end. No wonder it's gone viral. But in the rush for peak experiences, many people are skipping the foundational skills that would keep this kind of breathwork safe, and truly worth doing.

If you've tried a hyperventilation practice before, you've probably felt some kind of afterglow that feels nice. Moreover, for some, it's life-changing. While for others, it's overwhelming. And for many, it's novel but fleeting, leaving little behind. But for a growing number of people I see, it seems, this kind of breathwork leads to increased breathing dysfunction, increased anxiety, and an over-sensitized nervous system. (Good for my clinic business, maybe. But not the outcome I want to see.)

So what's happening during these over-breathing practices? In short: you're deliberately breathing way beyond your body's actual needs. More air in, more air out. Sometimes it's rhythmic and forceful and other times it's softer but continuous, cycling breath after breath without natural pauses.

Sessions can last a few minutes or stretch beyond thirty, even up to an hour and a half. Some methods include breath holds after deep inhales or exhales; others don't. The unifying principle is simple; you're flooding the system with air, dropping your CO_2 levels, and shifting your blood chemistry to impair oxygen delivery, on purpose.

In the short term, this causes dizziness, tingling, or even fainting. But in the long term? I'm convinced it can disrupt baseline breathing behaviours and chemistry if it's done without a solid foundation first.

There's also a mechanical issue. As most of these practices involve heavy mouth breathing, this bypasses your nose's natural filtration system. That means unfiltered, sometimes contaminated air heads straight for the vulnerable lower lobes of the lungs: Areas that aren't great at fighting off viruses or bacteria. Even healthy lungs can struggle to recover if pushed too far.

This mean these techniques are not appropriate for everyone, especially not as a casual, everyday wellness hack.

Hang on a minute, some of you may be thinking. Versions of these practices existed thousands of years ago in Taoist, Buddhist, and Yogic traditions... and they worked a charm. Surely they have a place?

Yes, I think you're right. But here's what those old masters seemed to understand: these techniques weren't for beginners. They weren't handed out like candy. They were reserved for specific purposes, taught with careful preparation, and often only shared with advanced students who had already built a stable physiological foundation.

Today, unfortunately, they're often marketed to everyone, with little attention to readiness, recovery, or risk.

So, should you try hyperventilating? Maybe. But if you do, do it smart. Personally, I use hyperventilation practices sparingly, maybe once a month, and only after checking that my baseline breath fitness is strong. I monitor my Breath Fitness Score (more on that in a moment), I pair any intense sessions with plenty of gentle recovery breathing, and I treat the practice like a supplement that's easy to overdose, not a core nutrient for everyday health.

Before diving into intense hyperventilation practices, it's essential to build your breathing baseline. At Breathe Your Truth, as you know, we call this your Breath Fitness.

If your daily breathing isn't strong, stable, and efficient, over-breathing won't transform you, it'll just send you down the path of more breathing dysfunction.

Use your Breath Fitness Score as your compass for what you can and shouldn't try.

Breath Fitness Score	How much hyperventilation?
0–50	Stick with the basics: Mindful low, belly breathing, and nasal breathing during daily activities. Build the foundation first BEFORE you try hyperventilation.
51-75	Light hyperventilation is okay, occasionally. Think only ten rounds (breath cycles) max. Always pair it with structured recovery. Most of your breathwork should focus on awareness and breathing *less*.
76-89	You can explore more intense practices. Sudarshan Kriya, or related practices fit. Just keep an eye on your BFS and make sure you're not slipping backward. Still, the bulk of your breathwork should emphasize breathing *less*.
90-100	Go for it. You've got the green light for full-on Wim Hof, Tummo, Holotropic, etc. But even now, *most* of your practice should center around gentle, breath-reducing techniques.

Now that you have a clearer sense of what you can safely experiment with, let's take a closer look at the different hyperventilation practices available.

When it comes to intentional over-breathing, a few techniques have stood the test of time and made their way into modern practice. Some of the oldest and most respected methods come from the yogic tradition of pranayama. Here are some of the most popular ones.

Bhastrika

One of the main players here is *Bhastrika*, often referred to as "bellows breath."

Bhastrika looks like rapid, active belly breathing, using forceful inhales and exhales. It's traditionally used to energize the system before meditation, essentially flipping the nervous system "on" before guiding it into deeper calm.

There are a few different styles of Bhastrika. Two versions that I particularly like, when done carefully, are the Bhastrika technique used within "Sudarshan Kriya," and a more controlled version called "Mukhya Bhastrika."

In Sudarshan Kriya, the Bhastrika phase involves sitting upright and coordinating strong breathing with arm movements. With each forceful inhale, the arms fly upward overhead; with each sharp exhale, the arms pull back down to the shoulders, fists closing tight. This pattern is typically repeated for three rounds of about twenty breaths, bookended by gentler, quieter breath practices that help settle the system.

Mukhya Bhastrika, on the other hand, is done from a kneeling, seated position. You hinge forward at the hips and blast out several sharp exhales through an open mouth, lips shaped in a small O, as you fold toward the ground. Once your forehead touches the floor, and your lungs are emptied, you pause for a few moments in silence. Then, you rise back up with a long, soft nasal inhale. After several rounds of this sequence, the real heart of the practice begins: resting in quiet, soft breathing. [100, 101]

In my view, this recovery phase isn't optional, it's essential. Without this quiet landing, the benefits of the practice are largely lost.

Rebirthing

Rebirthing breathwork was developed by Leonard Orr in the 1960s, inspired by elements of Tantric and Kundalini Yoga. [102] The core idea behind the method is bold, and it's that conscious breathing can help uncover and resolve deep-seated emotional wounds (especially those rooted in early childhood experiences).

The technique involves continuous, connected breathing with no pauses between the inhale and exhale. The goal is to maintain a relaxed, rhythmic cycle, allowing the breath to flow like an unbroken wave. It's usually done through the mouth. *You know how I feel about mouth breathing.*

Sessions often last twenty minutes or more and are typically facilitated by a guide. Proponents claim that Rebirthing can dissolve negative thought patterns and realign the mind with what they call "Universal Truth," a kind of innate harmony and happiness available beneath the layers of accumulated emotional debris. But to get there, most people suffer.

According to the principles of Rebirthing, the breather is encouraged to relive their trauma and to re-enter intense emotional states as a way of "working through it" and ultimately being "reborn."

While the intention might be healing, the reality can be incredibly risky, especially for people with PTSD, complex PTSD, or a fragile nervous system. This intense practice is probably best left to trained mental health professionals, not those with weekend, or even week-long, certification programs. Scientifically, the jury is still out on Rebirthing, even after all these years. Research has yet to consistently back up its sweeping therapeutic claims, which should leave anyone wondering: is such an extreme practice really necessary? I don't know.

Tummo Breathing

Tummo, meaning "inner fire" in Tibetan, is a traditional breathwork practice used by Himalayan monks for centuries to cultivate resilience against the brutal cold. Tummo combines deep, rhythmic over-breathing with extended breath holds, all while maintaining a strong visualization of inner heat building in the lower abdomen. [103, 104]

During the breath hold, practitioners engage an abdominal lock (known as a *bandha* in yogic traditions), intentionally contracting the core muscles to channel energy and concentrate heat around the navel region. It's not just theory, either; scientific studies have shown that skilled Tummo practitioners can raise their core body temperature by up to 14°F (about 7.8°C), even in freezing conditions. That's not small potatoes. It's a physiological feat that speaks to the incredible mind-body connection that breathwork can unlock.

Modern popular methods like the Wim Hof Method borrow heavily from Tummo's foundational concepts, specifically, the combination of over-breathing, breath retention, and mental focus. However, traditional Tummo isn't just a physical exercise. It's deeply embedded in spiritual training, involving meditation, visualization, and sometimes years of guided practice within a monastic community. In its original form, Tummo was less about biohacking and more about cultivating spiritual mastery. [105, 106]

Because Tummo involves intentional hyperventilation and strong internal muscle contractions, I recommend attempting it only if you already have a Breath Fitness Score of eighty-five or higher (and ideally with an experienced guide). Without a strong baseline of breath control, good CO_2 tolerance, and nervous system stability, the risks (including lightheadedness, panic, and dysregulation) can easily outweigh the rewards.

The Wim Hof Method

Now for one of the most controversial techniques of them all: The Wim Hof Method.

Wim Hof, often nicknamed "The Iceman," is an extreme athlete, performer, and self-identified research subject born 1959 in the Netherlands. He's most famous for his ability to withstand extreme cold, holding Guinness World Records for feats like swimming under glaciers and running a half-marathon barefoot above the Arctic Circle, all while regulating his breath and core temperature (for the most part).

The Wim Hof Method (WHM) rests on three pillars: breathwork, cold exposure, and mental focus (or in Hof's words, "commitment"). [105, 106] The breathing itself looks a lot like Tummo-inspired over-breathing (thirty to forty fast, deep breaths, followed by a breath-hold on an exhale for up to three minutes, then a shorter breath-hold after inhalation). This sequence is repeated several times.

Research into the WHM is a bit complicated because of the three pillars. The three pillars certainly add strength but also make it difficult to effectively control variables in a traditional research design. Regardless, the WHM has shown intriguing short-term effects on immune function, inflammation, and autonomic nervous system regulation. [107-109] It's not all snake oil; there's real science indicating that it can at least temporarily shift certain biological markers. That said, some of the bolder claims floating around (like curing cancer and reversing autoimmune diseases) haven't held up under rigorous, peer-reviewed scrutiny. [109]

And there is a much darker side to the WHM that is rarely discussed. His pursuits haven't come without cost. There are documented cases of health issues, including frozen corneas and hospitalizations after cold exposure. [110, 111] There are also, sadly, cases of accidental drowning linked to practicing this method. [112, 113]

Practitioners are now strongly warned not to practice near water, but the culture of bravado that sometimes surrounds this method, *push through the pain, be unstoppable,* makes accidents a predictable risk. A good dose of humility and common sense is non-negotiable here.

But to truly understand the WHM, you must understand the man behind it.

Wim Hof didn't surface this technique from a place of peak performance. He moved into it through crisis and desperation. After enduring unimaginable personal losses (including the death of his beloved wife to suicide) Wim Hof found himself trapped in overwhelming grief, pain, and on the verge of mental health collapse. [114] Breathing intensely, exposing himself to extreme cold, and pushing his body to its limits gave him a way out of his internal suffering. The WHM was born out of trauma: a way to survive unbearable emotional pain.

I suspect the majority of people today trying the WHM are not operating from the same place of survival. They're more simply over stressed, tired, or seeking personal growth. Applying such an extreme, shock-to-the-system method to a relatively healthy, functioning nervous system isn't saving them. And you could argue that for many, it's pulling their physiology down into survival mode unnecessarily – especially if they are not starting from a strong breathing foundation. And that's often leaving them more depleted than when they started.

Now, Wim Hof and his followers would likely be mortified, if not downright infuriated, by the suggestion that some people experience a net loss from this practice. And understandably so. That's clearly not his intention. In fact, it's quite the opposite. I'm simply speaking from clinical experience. Hyperventilation practices, when not balanced by solid breathing hygiene, tend to create problems. And let's be honest, most of us don't show up with excellent, or even decent breathing hygiene to begin with.

In other words: I think the Wim Hof Method (including cold exposure) is the right medicine for a very specific kind of wounding. But I don't think it's a tonic for everyday stress.

That's why I strongly recommend that anyone pursuing a regular Wim Hof Method practice have a solid Breath Fitness Score and monitor some relevant metrics over time to make sure they're experiencing a net gain.

Handle it with care. Respect the context it came from. And make sure you're using it for the right reasons: not just chasing a buzz or bragging rights.

Sudarshan Kriya

Sudarshan Kriya® is another breathwork phenomenon of our time, one that's gone global. Founded by Sri Sri Ravi Shankar in 1981 and taught through the Art of Living Foundation, this practice weaves together rhythmic breathing, movement, and meditation in a structured, methodical way. Its main goal is to reduce stress, anxiety, and emotional turbulence by changing the breath. [29, 115-120]

Unlike some hyperventilation methods that throw you straight into the deep end, Sudarshan Kriya takes a gentler, more scaffolded approach. The practice typically begins with a simple Yoga sequence to loosen up the body. Then comes chanting, designed to prime both breath and mind. Only after these preparatory steps does the more intense breathing phase begin: controlled rounds of seated, rhythmic over-breathing. The practice usually wraps up with a quiet meditation.

Even though this practice includes intentional over-breathing (and therefore falls under the hyperventilation umbrella) it's clear that significant care has been taken to guide practitioners both into and out of that state safely. That said, it still demands a certain level of breathing fitness (ideally, seventy-six or above) and self-awareness that many people simply don't have when they first encounter it.

In my clinical work, I've seen people who struggled with disrupted breathing chemistry after participating in Sudarshan Kriya. To be fair, the incidence is lower than with some other hyperventilation-heavy practices like Wim Hof. Still, some participants who initially felt fantastic reported that the benefits faded over time, replaced by subtle signs of respiratory imbalance, things like increased breathlessness, irritability, or a return of underlying anxiety.

My take? It's not that Sudarshan Kriya doesn't work. It's that many people step into it without the breathing foundation needed to truly benefit. If they'd spent some time first building their baseline, practicing resonant breathing, improving CO_2 tolerance, and refining their mechanics, I believe their outcomes would have been dramatically better.

If you're drawn to the yogic world and practices like this, Sudarshan Kriya can absolutely be a beautiful tool. I simply recommend adding about ten minutes of gentle resonant breathing into your daily routine for a few weeks beforehand. That alone can make a significant difference in how your system responds.

The bottom line is this: hyperventilation-based breathwork has a better chance of working if your breathing foundation is already solid. Build first. Then experiment wisely. These practices are powerful tools, not magic fixes. Like any supplement, when used intelligently, they can enhance your system. But if misused, they can easily tip the balance the wrong way.

Working Your Way Through the Breathwork Buffet

Okay, let's take a breath. That was a lot. There's an entire buffet of breathwork options out there, and it can feel overwhelming to figure out where to start.

But you don't have to guess. Just use your Breath Fitness score to guide you when it comes to breathwork, especially the hyperventilation stuff. So, if you haven't already, scan the QR code now to get your score. Or go to breatheyourtruth.com/score.

And a small but important reminder: Don't get pulled into thinking "more intense" means "more effective." Mastery comes from depth, not from chasing peak experiences. My educated guess is that you don't need bigger, harder, faster breathing. You, like most of us, need the opposite, even though the promise of peak experiences will always glitter at the edges.

Under-breathing practices, in my clinical experience, are where a lot of true healing and resilience begins. That doesn't mean you shouldn't explore everything you've learned here. You should. That's the gift of this journey: you now have the tools to experiment, to listen, to find what serves you best at each stage of your growth. But know this: there's no magic "healing" moment where the basics like low, slow nasal breathing stop mattering. They are and forever will be your bedrock practices, and they are not small.

They are everything.

Chapter 6:
Pulling It All Together

CONGRATULATIONS! YOU'VE MADE IT THROUGH the heavy-hitting concepts: the mechanics, the chemistry, and the mind-bending details of the psychophysiology of breathwork.

This next phase is about making breathwork personal and crafting a plan that fits your life.

Knowledge alone rarely creates change but application does. So, let's take a brief look at what we've explored so far and shape it into something practical.

The Triple M Triangle: An Overview

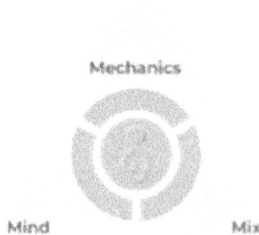

Mechanics

Mind   Mix

Breathing well starts with how the body moves. Specifically, how we create physical space for our breath.

This is the Mechanics section of our triangle. Proper Mechanics means releasing tension so that the diaphragm can come back online again and the breath can travel nice and low into the belly, but also into the sides, back, and lower ribs when you need it to.

This full range of movement is key because, even if you don't *need* to take a big, deep breath at any given moment, your body needs to know it can. When movement is restricted, the body sends out stressed-out warning signals: tightness, anxiety, fatigue. We want ease, flexibility and stability here so the breath can be effortless.

Then, we have the Mix part our our triangle. This orientates around your body's chemistry, that is, what your body does with the air you're breathing. Specifically, we're talking about CO_2, O_2 and nitric oxide (NO).

Here's where we pull back the veil on one of the most overlooked aspects of breathing. You learned that most of us breathe more than we need, and that affects our chemistry negatively. Breathing too much disrupts our CO_2 and blood pH balance, making us feel more restless, anxious, or fatigued than we should, especially during rest. Dialing back our breathing and allowing CO_2 levels to gently rise may not be intuitive, but it vastly improves our health.

The best and easiest way to do this is to train the body and mind to nose breathe softly and quietly, which helps optimize

CO_2 levels and boost NO production (our self-made anti-aging molecule, what a bonus!).

Then we came to the Mind segment of the triangle. This is where things got *really* fascinating (I hope). Given that the breath influences the mind, and the mind influences breath, this empowers us to take more ownership and authority over our mental health. Feeling worried and on-edge? You can adjust your breath to make you feel better. Feeling stuck in old breathing dysfunctions that come with anxiety? You can work on the mind to free up the breath.

In summary, we train the Mechanics to get the Mix just right, and we train the Mix to help set the Mind up for success, which in turn, nurtures good Mechanics… you get the picture. They're all interconnected and make up the foundation of healthy breathing.

All of this is interesting and empowering information to stew over, and you're already in a better position just by being aware of it all. A lot of the changes in your breathing will now spring forth from your unconscious mind, and before you know it, you'll be autocorrecting your Mechanics, optimizing your Mix and working on the Mind without even thinking about it.

But for those of you who prefer a nice, neat structure, a to-do list of sorts, here's where I'd begin to summarize it all in easy steps.

Step 1: Close Your Mouth and Nose-Breathe

If you do nothing else, do this. All the time. If you can.

If you're struggling to nose-breathe all the time, you could also spend a dedicated ten minutes each day focusing solely on nose breathing, like a meditation. Feel how the air moves through your nostrils, into the belly, and back out. Let it be slow, steady, rhymical, and smooth. It's worth investing a bit of extra time in this one at first, because it's by far the most powerful step towards reclaiming all three parts of the Triple M Triangle. If breathwork were a stock market, nose breathing would be your blue-chip investment, the one you never sell for anything else. It supports every pillar of the Triple M Triangle:

- Mechanics: Encourages opening of your (probably narrow and underused) nasal passages and promotes proper diaphragm movement
- Mix: Balances CO_2 levels and boosts nitric oxide for better oxygen delivery
- Mind: Stimulates the vagus nerve, calming the nervous system and flushing away stress

And maybe most importantly? It signals safety to your entire system.

Remember... mouth breathing is for survival. It's what your body does when you're running away from an angry cow or dodging an oncoming train. Nose breathing, on the other hand, says: "We're good. We're safe. All systems go."

The moral of the story is that unless you're sprinting for your life, you should be keeping the air flowing through your nose.

If you've been a mouth breather for a long time, this might feel tough at first, but the more you do it, the easier it gets. Once nasal breathing becomes your default during daily life, take it up a notch. Train yourself to stay nose-breathing during heavy exercise and physical stress. And if you want to go really crazy, tape your mouth shut before you go to sleep so you avoid mouth-breathing in your dreams. (More on the joys of mouth-taping to come, so stay tuned.)

And if you're still really struggle with it after trying your best? It's worth seeing an ENT specialist (an ear, nose, and throat doctor) to rule out structural issues. Note: these are very rare.

Your nose was made for performance. Train it well, and it'll pay dividends for life.

So go ahead and start policing yourself. Mouth breathing? Not on the menu. Not anymore.

Step 2: Breathe Deep, Not BIG

Now that you are nose-breathing like a pro, it's time to commence regular deep breathing.

BUT, and that's a huge but, that does not mean breathing *more*. Deep is not big, remember? As a general rule, we want to be inhaling very gently into the belly through the nose for about five seconds in, and five seconds out. About six breaths per minute. That's utilizing both deep breathing and Resonant Breathing, the subtle king of all breathwork techniques. You're wanting the kind of breath that naturally moves your belly out on the inhale, and in on the exhale.

You want this gentle ebb and flow to happen as much as possible (except during extremely intense physical exercise: pumping iron at the gym or swimming away from a great white shark). In general, there should be very few big gulps and gasps in your day-to-day. No erratic inhales. No exhales through the mouth unless you really need to. No filling the chest or the entirety of the lungs. There's no need for that. Think low, slow, smooth.

Sorry to harp on about it, but there really is a huge difference between a deep breath and a big breath. But most people confuse the two. Now, no judgment. A single, BIG breath can be useful. Refreshing, even. But it has to be deliberate. If you make a habit of breathing like that frequently, especially while you're sitting still, it can have some negative effects on your mind and body. You drop your CO_2 levels too low, overstimulate your nervous system, and unintentionally feed more anxiety into your life. [4, 6, 7, 10, 12, 68]

So go ahead: take that one deep breath if you need it. Let it clear the air. But don't chase it with ten more. Let your breath settle. Low. Slow. Smooth. That's the kind of breathing that helps you come back to yourself, especially when things get hard.

Step 3: Check Your Baseline and Breathe Accordingly

You're rocking the nose breathing, and you're habitually allowing the breath to rest low in the body. Effortless belly breathing is your game. The diaphragm is your right-hand man. *Low, slow* and *smooth* is your background mantra.

Once you're at this stage, it's time to retake your Breath Fitness Score test. Even if it's only been a couple weeks since you last took it, you should recheck your score. Why? Change happens faster than you might think when you start using your nose and diaphragm.

We're not just taking it out of curiosity either. This score can be super-helpful in guiding direction where you should and shouldn't go with more advanced breathwork practices.

If your Breath Fitness Score is between seventy-six and one hundred, that's your sign that your Mechanics, Mix, and Mind are solid enough to handle more intense breathwork. Although resonant breathing is my favorite and very low risk, I'm talking breath holding practices to build up your CO_2 tolerance, as well as a sprinkling of hyperventilation (if you so desire) like Bhastrika or Sudarshan Kriya, for example. The spicy stuff.

You might even experiment with Wim Hof's approach, if you feel the pull. Sometimes I do. Just make sure you balance your system afterwards. Spend twice as much time as you think you need on regulation practices like resonant breathing and CO_2 tolerance work to keep your system grounded and responsive. That is, practice breathing a lot *less* afterwards, comfortably, for the most part.

That said, I'd still proceed with caution and not go anywhere near the big stuff (hyperventilation) if you're not feeling your best. It's best to be firing on all cylinders before so profoundly messing with your chemistry.

I'll also encourage you *not* to practice big breathing or any kind of hyperventilation breathwork every day. You might end up undoing all the great work you've been doing up until now by screwing up your Mechanics, destabilizing your Mix and boggling your Mind! As I mentioned before, I wouldn't have a job were it not for people screwing up their day-to-day breathing through hyperventilation breathwork.

Whatever safe or crazy path you walk in the world of breathing, track something that reflects your breathing health.

Like, you guessed it, your Breath Fitness Score. Over time you'll see progress (or get the opportunity to course-correct if your score is decreasing).

Let's face it, life can get hard. And there are times when little good comes from terrorizing our breath with mysterious practices promising life-changing results. So, if those markers start slipping, that's your cue to slow down and reinforce your foundation.

Let your system regulate itself, don't aggravate it with hyperventilation. On the other hand, if your markers are trending in the right direction, and you feel good with the practices, you can keep playing.

But no matter what you do, make sure you stay friends with CO_2...

Step 4: Befriend CO_2

No matter how deep or how shallow you're hanging out in the breathwork rabbit hole, the fact remains true: in order to improve your body's chemistry, resilience, and performance, we are well served to work on tolerating higher CO_2 levels.

One way to do that is to consciously practice Resonant Breathing, mentioned in the second step: about five seconds in, five seconds out, through the nose, belly out, belly in. Smooth and gentle. If that feels too fast (I can hear many of you saying that), it's because your breath volume is too big. Think subtle (low volume), but still deep. And smile, at least internally. Do it as much as you can. But just ten minutes a day can make a huge difference.

But what can be even more effective, and give you results very quickly, is just getting used to breathing a bit less than you usually would during your day. This may sound vague, so let me give you some examples. You're reading a book, and you consciously breathe in a little less air and slow the exhale a bit. Not to an extent that you feel panic. Just enough that it feels "a little strange," but okay. It will become normal soon because it's actually how your body wants to breathe. You just have to shed a little maladaptive habit that your body got used (happens to the best of us).

And if you're running on a treadmill, or something like it, instead of opening your mouth, close it and breathe through your nose. Yes, your eyes will burn and snot will fly out your nose at first, but it changes. It gets better. You'll notice that you naturally slow the breath and take bigger longer breaths. This is exactly what you should do. This beautifully builds CO_2 tolerance as well as giving you a performance bump in two to three weeks of doing this.

The bottom line is: believe that CO_2 is your friend, not the bad guy, and work to have a little more of it in your body.

Step 5: Stay Consistent

Consistency beats intensity every time.

Rather than trying to master the entire multiverse of breathwork at once, getting obsessed with it, hammering it for a week then forgetting about it, focus on the foundations that you've learned so far. Commit to these four previous steps. Track your progress, and notice what changes mentally, physically, and emotionally.

This whole approach to "evolved" breathing is a marathon, not a sprint, and it's a process, not a destination. The gold at the "end" is just the gold you've picked up on the journey. Maybe that's true for life, too.

And the best part is, if you ever get lost, or you feel like life is pushing you two steps backward, you can always return to these simple foundations.

If you want to take your consistency a step further, (and are a fan of daily routines), yours could look a bit like this:

Morning (10 minutes)
Start the day by setting the tone:

- Sit, and watch the breath. First see what it's up to, then allow it to settle (if it's not already)

- Begin resonant breathing through the nose, using the diaphragm which means the breath feels like it's going deep in the belly (effortlessly). Five seconds in, five seconds out (low, slow, smooth, and subtle)
- If the urge arises, take a longer breath, your physiologic sigh, and enjoy a long luxurious breath out. Don't get greedy. Take one, then get back to being subtle

During the Day (As long as you like)

This is where the magic happens, right in the middle of daily life:

- Keep nose breathing during rest and activity (walking, working, cooking, exercise)
- Now and again, take a couple minutes to breathe a little less than usual and build that CO_2 tolerance (with the occasional two to three second breath hold)
- Try resonant breathing (five to six breaths per minute) while sitting and during light activities
- Take a "qi break" (as my friend Lee Holden calls it): five minutes of gentle Qi Gong to give your breath, body and mind the chance to do what they want to do... work together

Evening (10+ minutes)

Wind down and prep your nervous system for quality rest:

- Resonant breathing (still through the nose), this time a slightly shorter inhale (say, for four seconds), and a slightly longer exhale (say, for six seconds)
- Follow this with a couple of minutes of mindfulness meditation just noticing your breath, your body, or your thoughts without trying to change anything
- Aim to breathe through your nose during sleep (mouth taping might be your friend!)

This isn't about being perfect. It's about showing up daily and consistently. A few minutes here, a few there, and suddenly our breath starts working for you, not against you. Just a few minutes a day, woven through your routine, can create real, measurable change in how you think, feel, and move through the world.

Let your breath be the golden thread, the friend, that carries you through your days and your nights. Not just during your breathwork practice, but every other time in between, in the pauses, the quiet before sleep, the heat of a workout, or the emotion of a happy or really difficult moment.

This is where the practice becomes the lifestyle.

Chapter 7:
Breathing Metrics: The Love-Hate Relationship

LET'S GET THIS OUT OF THE WAY: breathing metrics aren't for everyone.

Some people love data. They light up at heart rate graphs, geek out on sleep trends, and can't wait to see their breathwork performance mapped out over time. Others? The idea of tracking anything feels like a fast track to burnout. If that's you, feel free to skip or skim this chapter. No shame. No pressure.

But for the data lovers... welcome to your playground.

So why should you consider tracking your breathing? Simply put, progress fuels progress. When you see a measurable shift, even a small one, it gives you a hit of happy chemicals and motivation that reinforces the habit. This is what psychologists call "self-efficacy": your belief that you can influence your own outcomes. And when you believe you can, you're far more likely to keep showing up. [121, 122]

It's worth mentioning, though, that metrics can also become a trap for some people. What starts as helpful feedback can spiral into perfectionism or self-judgment. If you're someone who's already deeply in tune with your body (able to feel when something's working or not) you might find the numbers distracting or redundant.

Still, I encourage even the most metric-averse among you to track one or two key markers. And one of those markers should be the Breath Fitness Score I've been blabbering on about during the course of this book. Not obsessively, just enough to catch trends every couple of weeks or so. Especially if you're incorporating more intense techniques like hyperventilation or intermittent hypoxic training.

So, get on your marks. And remember: the point isn't to get all-consumed by all this. It's to stay healthy and happy.

The 9 Metrics That Matter

Here's my list of the most meaningful metrics you can track, especially when breathwork becomes a regular part of your life.

The Breath Fitness Score (BFS)

The one I've been pushing hard (sorry, not sorry). This is your all-in-one snapshot of your Mechanics, Mix, and Mind. A small shift (say, from 53 to 57) is clinically meaningful. It's not a fastest-moving number, but it reflects deep, foundational change for the better. The ideal metric to aim for as a healthy human would be 76 and above.

Heart Rate During Activity

Your breathwork practice should make you more efficient physically. That means over time, your heart rate during exercise or stress should go down while your performance stays the same or improves. A 5 bpm drop while maintaining the same output is a great sign you're becoming metabolically and respiratory resilient. **The ideal metric to aim for as a healthy human in the age range of 35-40, for example, would be 125bpm for baseline work and 185bpm for intense intervals.**

Resting Heart Rate (RHR)

One of the clearest indicators of overall fitness. If your RHR is gradually dropping, that's your cardiovascular system saying, "Thanks for the upgrade." Even a 2bmp drop is worth celebrating. **The ideal metric to aim for as a healthy human would be 60bpm and below at rest.**

Breath Rate During Sleep

A slower, more stable breath rate while you sleep is a strong marker of parasympathetic activity (that rest, digest and repair mode your body needs to function well). Less breathing is better.

A two breath per minute drop during sleep is clinically significant. **The ideal metric to aim for as a healthy human would be 13 – 18 breaths per minute while sleeping.**

Timing of Your Lowest Heart Rate During Sleep

If your lowest HR occurs early in the night (the first third), it means you're dropping into deep, restorative sleep quickly. If it comes later in the night, it could indicate stress, poor recovery, or overstimulation.

Blood Pressure

If you have hypertension or blood pressure issues, breathwork can be a game-changer. Tracking it gives you real-world feedback on how your nervous system is responding to your new breathing habits over time. The goal is a downward trend, but *too* low, just like too high, can be a red flag. **The ideal metric to aim for as a healthy human would be approximately 115/80.**

End-Tidal CO_2 (ETCO$_2$)

This shows how much CO_2 is present at the end of your exhale. Essentially, it reflects how balanced your respiratory chemistry is. It's one of the most direct ways to measure your Mix. If you can access a capnography device (like the CapnoTrainer from Better Physiology), this data is gold. A 2-point change means progress. **The ideal metric to aim for as a healthy human would be 35 mmHg or higher.**

Heart Rate Variability (HRV)

Especially nighttime HRV. Higher HRV generally signals a balanced autonomic nervous system, better stress recovery, and improved adaptability. Breathwork can support this, but so can a lot of other things. It's a holistic marker. Sleep, stress, alcohol, illness, and exercise all affect HRV day to day. The trends, what makes it better or worse, matter more than the number itself. HRV is measured in milliseconds, and this number can vary significantly between individuals, but generally, a higher HRV is better.

Your Gut

How do you *feel*? Do you have more energy? Clearer focus? Better sleep? Your subjective experience matters just as much as the numbers. Don't ignore it. In fact, sometimes it's the most reliable metric of all.

Choosing a Device (Without Getting Overwhelmed)

You don't need lab-grade tools to get your metrics. Most consumer-grade wearables are good enough for identifying trends over time.

And don't panic over dips. One bad night doesn't mean your practice failed. For example, intense training (like breath holds or hyperventilation) might lower your HRV temporarily but offer long-term gains. Watch the weekly and monthly patterns, not the daily ups and downs.

Here are my go-to tools:

- Oura Ring & WHOOP Strap – Best for HRV, sleep, and long-term recovery trends

- Garmin & Apple Watch – Good for heart rate and fitness data

- Eight Sleep Mattress – Tracks sleep and auto-adjusts temperature (yes, please)

- Oxa – A wearable focused specifically on breath and biofeedback

- Breath Fitness Score Calculator – Free for you and our in-house tool at www.breatheyourtruth.com/score

- Pulse Oximeter – Crucial if you're exploring intermittent hypoxia or high-altitude protocols

- The CapnoTrainer® by Better Physiology. This is by far the most sophisticated and potentially useful piece of tech you can own if you're serious about improving breathing

An Extra Note on the CapnoTrainer®

For individual coaching, the CapnoTrainer can be an incredibly powerful tool. It allows for real-time monitoring of breathing patterns and helps identify which practices improve (or totally tank) your CO_2 levels.

While it's not designed for medical diagnosis, and its accuracy for determining absolute high or low CO_2 levels is moderate, it excels at what it was built for: education and training self-awareness.

Like many others, I've watched this feedback be incredibly valuable to my clients. The real benefit of this or any technology, though, is to support your ability to tune into your body more deeply, so you can eventually move beyond the screen and trust what you feel. Used wisely, the CapnoTrainer can fast-track that learning process.

That said, it's not for everyone. The CapnoTrainer is best suited to dedicated breath coaches or the committed client who's confident this tool will bring long-term value. If that's you, and you're considering getting one for yourself, go to www.breatheyourtruth.com/capnotrainer to learn more and check for any referred discounts.

Finding the Sweet Spot

When it comes to metrics, I'd advise tracking enough to stay informed, but not so much that you lose touch with your body.

For some people, tracking a handful of metrics keeps them inspired and motivated. For others, a once-a-week gut check works better.

The key is to make it support your practice, not overshadow it. And a gentle word of caution: if you're regularly practicing hyperventilation or pushing your chemistry through breathwork, I strongly recommend tracking these four metrics at minimum:

- Breath Fitness Score (especially the Max Breathlessness Test)
- Nighttime HRV
- Heart rate during light recovery
- Subjective energy and mood

These intense breathing practices can shift your physiology fast and without proper feedback, it's easy to overshoot.

So, track wisely.

Chapter 8:
The Politics of Mouth Taping

NOW THAT YOU KNOW HOW TO TRACK your breath and spot real progress, it's time to zoom into the finishing touches. You've officially reached the juiciest, most entertaining part of the book: the quirky, game-changing details that can take your breathing from "pretty good" to "life-altering." And we're kicking off with a controversial crowd favorite: mouth taping.

TikTok and other social media platforms are flooded with videos hyping the life-changing benefits of mouth taping, while others are out here trying to set the practice on fire with dire warnings of life-threatening dangers. [123]

Sleep medicine specialists, initially scoffing at the trend, have been scrambling to publish evidence-based commentary (some even reversing their initial disdain).

The earliest known advocate for mouth taping was Buteyko in the 1940s, [85, 124] but for decades, it stayed under the radar. That is, until now, when social media got its hands on it and turned it into the latest sleep hack.

The Science: Scarce but Growing

Recent studies suggest that, at a minimum, mouth taping can significantly improve obstructive sleep apnea, snoring, shortness of breath during activity, and bilevel ventilation (a non-invasive breathing machine that uses two air pressure levels to assist with breathing). [123, 125, 126][127, 128]

I know, I just pointed to studies offering some early support for mouth taping, even though they sit within a broader sea of expert opinion (and sleep industry bias) that leans against it. CPAP manufacturers? Definitely not fans. But here's the thing: I've seen it help people over and over again. So I'm taking a stand. Not because the science is settled, but because the results keep showing up. I'm betting my best roll of tape that time will land in favor of this simple but surprisingly powerful practice. To be fair, I completely agree with concerns raised in one study about mouth taping in people with severe soft palate obstruction, a relatively rare condition. In those cases, it could worsen airway flow. But for the vast majority, that risk is highly unlikely. And let's be honest: anyone with true obstructive issues will usually self-select out.

Rule number one of mouth taping? It has to make you feel better. Rule number two? Always use tape you can breathe through, just in case. For people who sleep with their mouths open (spoiler: a lot more people do than they realize), mouth taping can be a game-changer. For those who naturally sleep with

their mouths closed, there's no need. They try taping and feel...
nothing. No harm, and probably no benefit.

But for those who sleep on their backs, and those who tend to
mouth-breathe at night (most back sleepers do), or those who
struggle with nose breathing during activity, the difference that
comes with taping is massive. If you're one of those people, after
a week or two of mouth taping, you'll wake up feeling more
rested, more alert, and generally less like you just did twelve
rounds with a sleep demon.

Follow the protocol below and see how you feel. If you wake
up feeling *amazing*, no one will be able to convince you to stop.

Personally? I love waking up and still tasting toothpaste. It's a
weird but oddly satisfying perk.

If you want more than just *feelings* to go on, track your sleep
metrics. If mouth taping is your jam, you'll likely see
improvements in heart rate variability (HRV), total sleep time,
deep sleep, and REM sleep. Be your own scientist.

Despite all the benefits, mouth taping isn't for everyone, and
it's not for every situation. There are specific times when it's best
to skip it. Don't tape:

- If you're completely stuffed up with a cold: forcing nasal
  breathing when your nose is out of commission is just
  cruel. (But if you're just *slightly* congested, taping might
  actually help clear things up)

- If you've had a heavy night of drinking or are on strong sedatives
- If you have impaired heart or lung function or any condition that affects blood oxygenation – without the approval of your physician
- If you have a significant nasal or mid-face structural defect that makes nasal breathing difficult
- If you have allergies to tape or adhesives
- If the idea of mouth taping triggers anxiety

In the end, use good judgment. If it feels right, try it. If it gives you the creeps, skip it!

Picking the Right Tape

Let's get down to business: what kind of tape should you use? Will any old sticky tape do the trick? Should you just grab whatever's left over from last Christmas and slap it on your mouth like a festive science experiment? No. Please don't.

You want tape that's specifically made for skin. Not duct tape. Not packing tape. Not scotch tape. Seriously.

Go for something gentle, skin-safe, and ideally hypoallergenic. Dynamic tape usually works great. Crucial tip: press it onto the back of your hand first to tone down the stickiness. Otherwise, when you peel it off in the morning, you might take a layer of lip with it and spend the rest of the day explaining why your mouth looks like it lost a fight with a sandblaster. And, we want it less sticky so if your body isn't liking it, you can open your mouth and breathe.

Some solid tape choices would be:

- Dynamic Tape (Kinesio Tape® is a decent brand)
- Hypafix® or Cover Roll®
- Somnifix®
- Myotape by Oxygen Advantage
- 3M® Micropore Tape

How to Ease Into It (The Protocol)

Mouth taping should be a *suggestion*, not a *demand*. That means using a tape that allows you to open your mouth if needed. You don't want to wear tape that you have to use your hands to remove. You should be able to just "open your mouth," with a little force to break through it.

Another tip: Fancy donut-shaped tapes (with a hole in the middle) are great. They gently encourage nasal breathing but still allow for mouth breathing if necessary. Remember, the tape doesn't need to seal your entire mouth shut (and probably shouldn't). The goal is just to give your body a gentle reminder to keep your lips closed. A less fancy approach is to use a thin vertical strip, right down the center of your lips. About an inch wide is usually enough to nudge your brain without irritating your skin or your sense of dignity.

Once you've purchased your tape, remember:

1. Start slow – before taping your mouth, press the tape onto the back of your hand first to remove excess adhesive

2. Remove it gently – don't rip it off like a band-aid unless you enjoy pain

3. Test drive it – tape up while reading or working on the computer for thirty minutes. No problem? Move to step 4

4. Light activity – wear it while doing low-key tasks like folding laundry or vacuuming. Still easy? Next step

5. Try it at night – *gradually*. Most people need two to three nights before they can sleep through the night with tape on. If it interrupts sleep, take it off. No point in losing sleep trying to sleep better

Before we sign off on sleeping hacks, there's another secret weapon that is probably worth mentioning for those of you who's jaw falls backward when you sleep: Mandibular Advancement Devices (MADs). This, combined with mouth taping, may well be the hack of the century for you open-mouthed snoozers.

These are hilarious looking contraptions you put over your head and secure below your chin. They're surprisingly comfortable, though. They gently push your lower jaw forward while you sleep. Why? Because this keeps your airways even more open, reducing snoring and sleep apnea shenanigans.

Don't Just Stop at Better Sleep

Want to improve physical performance? Once you've conquered mouth taping during sleep, the next door swings wide open: taping your mouth during exercise.

I know. It sounds intense. But hear me out: nothing will keep you more honest about your breathing than a little piece of tape. Start easy. Walk, spin lightly, stroll on a treadmill. Then, as your tolerance grows, keep taping during more strenuous sessions.

Why bother? Because taping during movement transforms how your body performs under pressure. It helps build CO_2 tolerance, which not only improves your baseline breathing but also your ability to buffer lactic acid during intense exertion. It also keeps you in a parasympathetic state longer, anchoring your nervous system in calm, even as your body works hard. You stay grounded, present, and in control.

At the same time, it helps shift the breathing down into the diaphragm, taking strain off your neck, shoulders, and upper chest. Your center of gravity then lowers, helping you move with more coordination and stability.

And believe it or not, your body will probably look better doing it. There's something unmistakably graceful about someone who moves with calm, grounded breath.

While you're on the fork, another fork may appear. At some point (sooner than you think), you'll probably hit it: the moment where nasal breathing feels like it just isn't enough. You'll feel the pull to rip the tape off, open your mouth, and gulp air like a trout on a dock.

In this case, you have two choices:

Option A: Switch to the lesser of two evils: breathe in through your nose, out through your mouth.

Option B: Stay 100% nasal... even if it means slowing down or resting

Which one creates change faster? Option B. Every time. I've seen this play out dozens of times. Right around the three-week mark, the magic of your nasal-breathing commitment happens:

- Performance improves
- Heart rate drops
- Recovery improves
- Nasal breathing feels natural (and sometimes better than mouth breathing ever did)

That's the threshold. Once you cross it, everything shifts.

Crossing the nasal breathing tolerance barrier can get messy. As you push your limits and resist the urge to mouth-breathe, snot may start flying out and your eyes might burn and water. This reaction is likely due to cortisol and adrenaline acting as natural antihistamines, clearing out congestion. Not pleasant, but believe it or not, you *want* this stage. It's a sign that you're making real anatomical changes to your nasal passages. You're transforming thick, boggy, half-clogged airways into sleek, ninja-like breathing channels.

Over time, this process won't just improve airflow, it will slowly remodel the internal bony diameter of your nasal passages for the better.

What Happened to Ray and I

My friend and colleague Ray lived all this firsthand.

We were working with a patient together when he heard me talk about this fork in the road, and inspired, Ray decided to try it himself. He committed to nasal breathing on his brutal West Hills bike commute in Portland, Oregon. (Think serious hills.)

At first? Not enjoyable. But Ray did the right thing and geared way down. He slowed his pace but stuck to breathing through his nose. And sure enough, around the three-week mark, he crossed the line: super steady climbs. No mouth breathing. And, bonus, he was stronger than before. Ray was sold. Today, he teaches the same progression to his own patients at Wildwood Physical Therapy in Portland.

My own story echoes the same mantra: stick with it. Years before Ray did, I taped my mouth shut twice a week in spin classes (the ones I *took*, not the ones I taught). It was brutal for two weeks: snotty nose, burning eyes, serious willpower tests. Then, threshold crossed. Not only did nasal breathing feel so good, but my power shot up from an average of 170 watts to 230 watts per ride all nasal, all day. What an awesome feeling! And it's waiting for you too if you're willing to stay the course.

How Long Should You Tape For?

Some lucky folks only need to tape for a couple of months before their body "gets it" and starts keeping the mouth shut on its own both during sleep and exercise. If you're one of those, feel free to dial it back whenever you're ready.

I've got no problem staying nasal during exercise, so I don't tape at the gym. But sleep? That's another story. Even after ten years trying, I still catch myself mouth breathing at night. I'm a back-and-side sleeper, and apparently, my body refuses to take the hint. So, I still tape. Maybe I'm just stubborn by nature, but I know I'm not alone. If that's you too, welcome to the long-haul crew. Bottom line is, you'll have to experiment and see what works best for you. You won't regret it.

Chapter 9:
Build Your Anxiety Shield

IF I COULD WAVE A MAGIC WAND and erase the biggest roadblock to happiness and optimal breathing, it would be anxiety. But, since I have yet to acquire any magical powers (still working on that), we've got to tackle this one the old-fashioned way: methodically, strategically, and with the sincerest of good intentions.

But before we dive into your anti-anxiety breathwork toolkit, let's check off some general health items to set us up for success.

Step 1: Get Your House in Order (At Least a Little)

A great place to kickstart supporting your wellbeing is with therapy.

Think of it as a personal trainer for your inner world. You don't need to be falling apart to benefit from therapy. Just having a pro help you navigate life's weirdness is a gift.

Then there's what you eat. Choose meals that make you feel good long-term, not just for the ten minutes after you inhale that donut. Highly processed foods, sugar, and low-quality fats mess with your nervous system. You don't have to be perfect, but nourishing your brain and body helps you feel calmer and more resilient. Aim for whole, nutrient-rich foods. Think quality proteins, healthy fats, and carbs that grow from the earth. Eating seasonally and locally supports both your body and internal rhythms.

My favorite resources are Mindful Eating by Marc David, Fiber Fueled by Dr. Will Bulsiewicz, and Good Energy by Dr. Casey Means.

While we're taking pot-shots at the "fun" stuff, let's talk about alcohol and drugs. Look, I get it. Having a drink or two can be a powerful reminder that we're meant to feel good. But over time, alcohol and recreational drugs chip away at your brain's natural ability to regulate anxiety. I know, I know… inconvenient truth alert. Sorry for bringing it up. (But also… not sorry.)

If you're feeling overwhelmed, cutting back might be the unexpected fix you didn't know would work. Reducing alcohol and drugs will also have a positive effect on your sleep. That brings us nicely onto the next point.

Poor sleep = more anxiety. No surprise. If you're struggling with sleep, make it a priority to fix it. Not in a "someday" kind of way, but now. Better boundaries with screens, consistent sleep times, even mouth taping, whatever helps you get real rest. And don't forget to stock up on more morning light, and less evening light.

Your body wants to sync with the sun. Morning light tells your brain it's go-time. Dim evening light helps you wind down. Wake at the same time every day (yes, weekends too), and get sunlight in your eyes within the first hour of waking up. Cloudy day? Stay out longer. *The Circadian Code* by Dr. Satchin Panda is a brilliant resource on this topic.

And last but not least – the most heartfelt nudge I'll provide: move your body. Exercise is just as much for your *mental health* as your physical health. Moving your body regularly helps regulate stress hormones, improves sleep, boosts brain chemistry, and keeps your nervous system on more stable ground. [129-134]

You don't need to train for a marathon or crush high-intensity workouts every day. Just move for no reason. Walk. Dance. Stretch. Lift something heavy. Shake it out. Even better? Try to move at consistent times of day – don't wait for divine inspiration that may or may not show up. Be on a schedule. Consistency, precision, and intention beat intensity every time, and this builds trust (aka patterns) in the nervous system. Your future, less-anxious self will thank you.

Movement, and everything else you've learned in this section, is medicinal when it comes to treating anxiety and boosting our wellbeing. If you'd like to get a snapshot of your overall health and where you're at with your wellbeing, you can take the Breathe Your Truth Wellness Questionnaire. It's free. Go to www.breatheyourtruth.com/wellness to check it out.

Once you've handled the basics, or at least acknowledged them, it's time to unlock one of the most powerful anxiety-regulating tools you already own: your breath.

Step 2: Your Anti-Anxiety Shield: The Breathwork Toolkit

No prescription. This is a built-in system, always available, always ready to help regulate your nervous system. The tools that follow can be used as standalone practices or done in the sequence provided for a power packed practice.

Tool 1: Quiet Breathing

Anxiety tends to hijack our breath, making it faster, shallower, and higher in the chest. That's why quiet breathing is tool #1. It might sound simple, but done well, it makes a huge difference. Here's what makes it so effective:

a. Nasal

Nose breathing calms the brain, encourages better diaphragm use, and filters and humidifies the air. It's foundational for nervous system regulation. Make it your default, even during exercise.[30, 75, 130-145]

b. Low in the body

Let the breath drop into the lower belly. Don't force it, just get out of the way. Let gravity and relaxation do the work.

c. Slow

This will happen naturally when you breathe low and quiet. But here's the magic trick: slow down the *start* of your exhale, just a bit. That moment is golden. It stimulates the vagus nerve and invites your system into a more grounded, relaxed state.

I'm still waiting to see this level of exhale specificity emerge in scientific literature. But clinically, while monitoring heart rate variability and CO_2 levels, I see it again and again: the biggest shifts happen with this simple adjustment in the very beginning of the exhale.

Try it for yourself. Compare slowing the *beginning* of your exhale versus the middle or tail end. Most people can literally feel their heart rate start to settle when they slow the start, something that doesn't happen as easily later in the exhale.

Tool 2: The Physiologic Sigh

One of the quickest ways to shift gears from stress to calm is a technique called the "physiological sigh," popularized by Dr.

Andrew Huberman. It's a two-part inhale followed by a long exhale.

First, take a deep breath in through your nose, then sneak in a second, smaller sip of air right on top. That second breath helps pop open the little air sacs (alveoli) in your lungs, giving them more surface area to release carbon dioxide. Then follow it up with a slow, extended exhale.

Want to get even more? Remember to slow down the start of that exhale for reasons stated above. I'm so sure that's where the vagus nerve and the parasympathetic nervous system get their strongest cue to ramp up. It's like pressing a soft internal reset button; it's quiet, powerful, and fast-acting.

Yes, I know that up to now I've been telling you to avoid taking big breaths and filling your lungs to the brim, but this is an exception and it's only *one* breath.

Tool 3: Hum

Just a few minutes of soft humming can increase nitric oxide levels in the nasal passages (hello, better circulation and oxygen uptake), while also stimulating the vagus nerve, your nervous system's balancing switch. The trick is to keep it gentle and relaxed. Here's the nuance: put more emphasis on the "h" than the "m." Think of it like a whispered hum "hhhhhhhhmm" rather than a forced, buzzy drone. That "h" gently opens the back of the throat, creating space and triggering one of the vagus nerve's key connection points. Start with just a few minutes. No straining. No big inhales.

Tool 4. Resonant Breathing

Now we focus on the timing of your inhales and exhales. Try inhaling through your nose for five to six seconds. Then try exhaling for the same amount of time. Five in, five out. Or six in, six out.

This breath improves your heart rate variability, and that helps regulate stress and calms you down. You can use this as a first-aid tool, but you should also get consistent with this. Try ten minutes in the morning and ten minutes before bed. Give yourself a week before you make a judgment call on this practice. It's simple, but potent.

If your goal is relaxation, make the exhale a little longer than the inhale. If your goal is to stay alert, focused, and calm, keep the inhale and exhale even.

Tool 5. Alternate Nostril Breathing (Nadishodhana)

If you want to ramp things up a little, that's where alternate nostril breathing comes in. It's been around for a couple of thousand years, and it works just as well today as it did for the ancient, chilled-out yogis. Nadishodhana, a classic pranayama practice, has a solid body of evidence behind it, especially for improving heart rate variability and reducing anxiety. [76, 77, 138, 140, 141, 146-156]

Here's how to do it. Breathe along with me right now:

- Sit upright and hold this book with your left hand
- Bring your right hand to your nose
- Block your right nostril with your thumb and inhale through the left
- Block your left nostril with your ring finger, release your thumb and exhale through the right
- Inhale through the right nostril, then block it with your thumb again
- Exhale through the left
- Inhale through the left
- Block it
- Exhale through the right
- Inhale through the right
- Block it
- Exhale through the left
- Inhale through the left
- Block it

- And repeat for ten minutes

And if you're too anxious to get your head around this? Just block the right nostril and breathe in and out of your left nostril only. Do this for ten minutes.

But What About Panic Attacks?

Now let's talk about the extreme end of anxiety. Panic attacks.

I'd be remiss not to share what I've learned through experience, both personal and professional, about supporting someone (or yourself) in the middle of a full-blown panic attack.

First things first: use the tools above.

If you feel a wave of panic building, or if you're already caught in it, go straight to your anti-anxiety breathwork toolkit. Start nasal breathing, if you can. Slow your inhales and exhales, if possible. Try a physiological sigh, humming, resonant breathing or alternate nostril breathing, if you're able. Just try your absolute best to control your breathing and slow down the hyperventilation. That's all you can do.

But here's the honest truth: sometimes, even when you do everything right, nothing seems to work fast enough. And that's okay.

Panic can be slippery and irrational. It can override even the most solid breathwork techniques or nervous system hacks. That doesn't mean they're not working, it just means the storm is loud. Sometimes, the best you can do is ride it out while keeping one hand on the railing.

Do you. I've known people who cope with panic attacks in very unique ways, some need to sprint, punch the air, or lift weights like their life depends on it. And honestly? That can help. Intense movement raises CO_2 levels and can chemically shift your state. So if you need to move, move, move.

But the long-term goal is to build the capacity to soothe your system without needing to engage in extreme coping mechanisms. And if you build your anxiety shield up by using all the tools provided to you in this chapter, with a bit of luck, and a lot of patience, panic attacks will become a very rare occurrence for you.

And if I ever stumble across a foolproof method, I promise, I'll write another book.

The Final Word on Anxiety and Breath

If you take nothing else away from this, know this: your breath is a built-in remote control for your nervous system.

Shallow, fast breathing? Triggers anxiety.

Slow, low breathing? Signals safety and calm.

Your breath is the easiest, most accessible way to tell your body it's safe. And when you combine it with smart lifestyle choices, you're building a rock-solid anxiety shield.

Activity 5: Build Your Anxiety Shield

Let's work through this together. Join me for a guided video routine in Activity 5: Build Your Anxiety Shield, where we'll practice the breathing techniques from this chapter step by step. Visit breatheyourtruth.com/breathwork-exposed or scan the QR code below to get started.

Chapter 10:
Supercharging Your Workout

ARE YOU CRUSHING YOUR WORKOUTS, or are they crushing you?

If you're walking out of the gym feeling like you just got steamrolled, something's off. And no, the answer isn't just "work harder." The trick is to work smarter. And the shortcut to that is, you guessed it, your breath.

How you breathe in the gym determines how you breathe the rest of the day (and even at night). If you're panting, holding your breath, or gasping at the gym, you're training your body that it's okay to do that all the time.

That's problematic for your breath mechanics as well as the chemistry of your blood, and it sends your nervous system on an involuntary roller coaster ride.

But if you master your breath? You'll need *less* effort to get bigger gains, feel less wrecked, and even recover faster. Sounds like magic, right? Well, it's not. It's science.

Let's start from the very beginning.

Warm-Up: Don't Let Your Breath Get Ahead of You

Warm-ups aren't just about getting loose and preparing your body for movement; they're about prepping your mind and your breath too.

But most of us start over-breathing during our warmups, and this preps the body perfectly for under-performance during our actual workouts. It's like the mind knows what is coming and triggers bigger breathing way sooner than needed. This over breathing dumps too much CO_2, trapping oxygen just when you want this opposite to happen. You want a gentle build-up of CO_2 because it sets up your body for better performance.

Solution? Pay attention to your breath when you warm up. The simple act of noticing it helps steady it. Keep it light, smooth, and steady. No huffing and puffing yet (or ever), just chill, even as you warm up. Nose breathing only. It makes you more efficient, keeps your breath lower in your body, and floods your lungs with nitric oxide, which helps oxygen absorption.

Strength Training: Flip Your Breathing Script

Strength training is designed to get you to build muscle and gain strength through lifting weights. And your breath is going to help you do it faster and better.

Here's where things get wild. Most people are taught to exhale when they push or lift, but I'm going to suggest the opposite:

slowly exhale on the return or lowering phase instead. This is called the "eccentric phase," when the muscle is lengthening under tension.

Why flip it? For one, exhaling during the eccentric phase taps into greater core stability. And I don't just mean your abs, I'm talking about the deep team players: your pelvic floor, transversus abdominis, and multifidus. These muscles light up more effectively on the exhale, giving your spine and nervous system a rock-solid foundation. [38, 157-162]

There's also a strength benefit. Muscles tend to grow stronger more efficiently when we slow down and control the eccentric part of a movement. By pairing that with a slow, stable exhale, you're essentially doubling down, building more strength than you would doing it quickly with an inhale. And this way, you can lessen the weight. Bottom line? Less weight, more gains, fewer injuries.

And maybe the most overlooked benefit? Nervous system regulation. When you slow your exhale, especially by controlling the eccentric phase, you keep your parasympathetic system engaged. That's your rest-and-digest mode, sure, but it's also your *think clearly, learn efficiently, and feel great* mode. It's worth training into your body. That's not just helpful during workouts, it teaches your system how to stay calm, focused, and composed when life throws you a curveball.

Example: Bench Press

- Inhale while pressing up – feeling your kidney area or lower ribs expanding into the bench. Don't forget nose breathing
- Exhale slowly while lowering the weight slowly (nose or mouth is okay, but nose is better)

Example: Lat Pulldown

- Inhale while pulling down. Remember your kidneys and nose
- Exhale slowly while slowly releasing back up

Take notice of how you feel after a few activities done this way. I advocate that you will feel less spinning, energy up in your head, and more grounded, centered, and in control. It's a great feeling. Train this feeling in the gym and it show up more in your day.

Power Training: Unleash the Beast

This is where things get explosive. Power training is all about fast, high-intensity movements. Think sprints, box jumps, Olympic lifts, or anything that requires maximum effort in minimum time. It's not about grinding through reps slowly, it's about speed, force, and intention.

And here, we return to the classic breathing strategy: a sharp, forceful exhale on the effort. Why? Because in power training, the goal is simple: get from point A to point B as fast and forcefully as possible.

A strong exhale helps the diaphragm contract quickly, syncing your breath with the explosive demand. It also clears CO_2 faster, making space for the lactic acid that inevitably builds up during intense output.

Just as importantly, it ramps up your nervous system on purpose. Instead of letting stress hijack you, you're shaking things up deliberately, putting your body into a high-alert state to meet the challenge.

Power training is usually a small but vital part of an overall fitness routine. Unless you're training specifically for athletic performance (like sprinting, throwing, or jumping), it might make up around twenty percent of your weekly training. [163] These sessions teach your system to tolerate intensity, recover quickly, and respond with precision under pressure.

Remember, this is the beast-mode part of your training, and your breath needs to match the energy.

Example: Kettlebell Swing

- Inhale during the hinge phase as the kettlebell swings back between your legs. Feel the breath drop into your lower ribs and back body
- Sharp, forceful exhale through the nose or mouth as you drive your hips forward and launch the kettlebell up. Let the breath match the snap

Example: Jump Squat

- Inhale as you lower into the squat position, steady and grounded through the nose, filling the lower ribs and preparing for launch
- Explosive exhale through the mouth as you push off the ground and jump. Let the breath support the lift and fire up your nervous system

This method turns you into a powerhouse while keeping you efficient. You get to access all your chips in a strategic way.

Ab Work

Most people do ab exercises with sharp, explosive breathing: a quick exhale on the crunch, a gasp of air on the way down. But there's a different, more intentional way to breathe that regulates your system instead of ramping it up. Here, we keep our movements and our breathing more separate.

Try this: breathe at a steady rhythm while doing your ab work, five seconds in, five seconds out. If that feels too long, shorten to three or four seconds. It's not meant to make the workout harder; it's meant to help you stay calm, focused, and steady.

As we learned in Chapter 4 on the mind, this pace puts you around six breaths per minute, which is a sweet spot for improving heart rate variability and overall nervous system control.[164] It brings your awareness back online and starts the cool-down process before the workout is even over.

It also reduces unnecessary tension. When you regulate your breath, you stop wasting energy in places that don't help (like your face). Most people scrunch their face and strain their neck when working hard. But when you focus on your breath, those habits fade. Try it both ways. You might laugh at the face you make when you're not breathing mindfully.

Example: A Simple Crunch (kind-of connected breath)

- Do three to five short-range crunches during a single inhale. Then three to five on a single exhale

Example: A Simple Crunch (disconnected breath)

- Keep your breath slow and steady, in and out, while doing crunches at a comfortable rhythm. The breath and the movement are completely separate

Both approaches are useful. Connecting the breath to the movement helps you isolate and strengthen the muscle. Disconnecting it helps your nervous system stay calm and steady, even as your body moves. I usually connect my breath about seventy-five percent of the time and consciously disconnect the other twenty-five percent. Both are skills worth training.

Stretching: The Breath-to-Flexibility Connection

Ever catch yourself holding your breath during a stretch? Most people do. But that breath-hold sends the wrong message to your nervous system. It tells your body that something's wrong, so your muscles brace instead of release. And if you carry that same pattern into the rest of your day, you're walking around like a tightly wound spring.

Your breath and your muscle tension are directly linked. A calm, steady breath says, "You're safe," and when your body feels safe, it lets go.

So, how do you stretch smarter?

Hold each stretch for four to ten slow, steady breaths. This gives your nervous system time to register safety and override the stretch reflex (the body's built-in safety mechanism that resists lengthening to prevent injury). That reflex usually takes about thirty seconds to calm down, which lines up almost perfectly with five or six long breaths. If you rush or force it, your muscles just fight back. If you breathe through it, they start to melt.

Cool-Down: Make Gains for Free

Let's be real, most people skip the cool-down, or just do a couple of half-hearted stretches and call it good. But a proper cool-down is essential for recovery. And your breath can be one of the most powerful tools to support it.

When you cool down, you're teaching your nervous system that it can go hard and then come back to calm with you in the driver's seat. Gentle movement after intense effort can also help flush out lactic acid and other byproducts more effectively than simply flopping on the floor and hoping for the best. It also keeps circulation going and speeds up the cleanup crew. [165]

I have a theory on this. You've probably heard Newton's first law, "objects in motion stay in motion." Well, your nervous system probably works the same way. After a workout, everything's still running hot: elevated heart rate, fast breathing, heightened brain activity. If you don't guide your system back down, it can stay revved for hours, whether you want it to or not.

Here's how I suggest you do it:

- Stay in motion after your workout. Keep moving at low intensity (walk, bike, treadmill)
- Focus on breathing through your nose, and let the breath be slow, and low, as soon as possible
- Bonus/luxury end: Lay down for full recovery. Find a spot, lie on the floor or earth. Let everything settle

This simple process resets your nervous system fast, prepping you for better recovery and future performance.

Final Takeaway

Next time you step into the gym, remember: your breath is your secret weapon. Mastering it means building strength more efficiently, using less weight for better results, feeling more energized during and after your workout, and recovering faster so you can perform even better next time.

Train your breath like you train your body, and watch everything level up.

Scan the QR code for an on-demand mini-course and real-time workout demonstrations to bring it all to life. Or, go to breatheyourtruth.com/gym to find out more.

Chapter 11:
Swimming: The Breathwork Truth-Teller

SWIMMING IS BREATHWORK'S ULTIMATE truth-teller. In the water, you either control your breath and learn from it, or it controls you. There's nowhere to hide.

And that's exactly why I love it. Every time you swim, you are training your breath for better or worse. Whether you mean to or not. So, let's make sure that training is intentional, intelligent, and actually serving you. Whether you're an elite swimmer chasing milliseconds or an average Joe just trying to survive your local lane swimming session, this is your chapter.

What Goes Wrong in the Water?

There a few cards stacked against awesome breathing in the water... unless you were born with gills.

The first is that you're going to be forced to mouth-breathe. Now, if you've read the rest of this book, you'll know I've been relentless about avoiding mouth breathing. But swimming is the big exception. When your face is in the water and you have a split second to inhale with water streaming down your face, your mouth is the only answer.

Try it (don't try it) with your nose. You'll feel like water just shot into your brain. And that's not good. So, unless you're truly swimming with your face out of the water (which I do not recommend), you'll need to breathe in through your mouth. We're going to discover other ways to achieve a net breathing gain by playing in the water soon. But first, let's finish the picture of tricky things swimmers must overcome.

Next, the overhead arm position in swimming tends to encourage upper chest breathing. Add the short, fast, choppy breaths mixed with frequent breath holds and it's easy to see how swimming can program some pretty dysfunctional patterns into your system.

Lastly, there's the pressure, the subtle kind. Watching the clock. Trying to keep up with your lane. Performing for a coach. None of this is bad in absolute terms, but it frequently becomes bad because we internalize or prioritize external reward and opinion as being more important than what we feel or learn from ourselves.

Before you know it, the swim becomes more about survival or performance for someone else instead of a healthy, awareness-building exercise. You may have guessed this by now, but that external focus frequently leads to what we might accurately describe as "anxiety breathing." And we train ourselves into breathing like that outside the pool.

But wait, don't turn in your Speedos and goggles quite yet. There's the twist. The cards stacked in your favor are powerful. If used skillfully, swimming can lead to a huge net gain in your overall breath fitness.

Because you're not breathing as frequently, swimming naturally limits air intake. This gives you an opportunity to build tolerance to CO_2: the key marker of better breathing chemistry. And when your CO_2 tolerance improves, so does oxygen delivery, and your lactic acid tolerance. [166, 167]

Translation: you can swim faster, with less suffering.

Maybe even more profound is the opportunity to stay aware of your breath. When you're swimming and consciously tuning in, it's one of the best ways to anchor yourself in the present moment. And what lives in the present? Peace and happiness (eventually, if not immediately). You quiet the mind, reduce rumination, and increase your capacity for focus both in and out of the pool.

We'll cover specifics in the pages ahead, but here are some big picture tips to get you started:

- Welcome mild air hunger during swim sets. This is your CO_2 tolerance training, and it's worth it
- Stay aware of your breath while swimming. Awareness alone is a powerful way to win the mental game of swimming

- Watch for the drift into external performance mode. It's okay to track your time and push yourself but don't lose the conversation with your breath in the process

Yes, it might feel uncomfortable at first. But that discomfort pays dividends. Every moment you spend being fully present with your breath is a win. And those wins add up. Trust me, I know.

The Over-Breathing Swimmer

Back when I was a competitive swimmer in college, training hard, swimming fast, and performing at my physical peak, you'd think I'd be a master of breath control. But I was much better at holding my breath as a twelve-year-old than I was at twenty-two, and at the height of my swimming career.

I couldn't make sense of it at the time. How could I be a fitter, stronger, more experienced swimmer, and somehow have gotten worse at breath holding?

I get it now. As my career progressed, so did the pressure. While I loved swimming in college, every workout felt like a threat to my existence. Don't get me wrong, the practice pool was exciting: fast swimmers, big water, and huge energy. But underneath all that? Anxiety. Anxiety that I wasn't going to be able to keep up with the pool. It doesn't make sense looking back, because while I was not the fastest, I was far from the slowest at

Bemidji State, and later the University of Wisconsin-Madison. I was just fine. I was at the level that most of the workouts were written for. But over time, I built a story of fear and anxiety that lived on its own terms in my body without my permission. And it changed my breathing.

Stress is not necessarily bad, especially this kind of stress. What makes it good or bad is what is done with it. It this case, if I could have leveraged the adrenaline surging pre workout anxiety for better performance during the workout, then developed the skill of bouncing back to a strong parasympathetic dominated state after training. I'm confident I wouldn't have messed up my breathing if I were having a bit more fun while I was swimming and relaxing a bit more afterward.

But as it was, I hardwired over-breathing into my system. I took more breaths than I needed by paying very little attention to my breathing. And eventually, after training my hindbrain to be overly sensitive to carbon dioxide, I started to physiologically feel like I needed more breaths. It wasn't just behavior, now it was also my physiology. I got stuck.

It didn't matter how many laps I swam or how fit I was becoming. My breath mechanics were quietly getting worse, and my neck, back and shoulders started hurting. It took me years to figure out why. But once I did, it took a lot less time to start undoing it.

Decades after my college career, I started focusing less on the clock, less on the pressure to keep up with the lane and let go of the need to prove anything to anyone. I brought in simple breathing practices, some of which you'll learn in this chapter. It took equal parts breath practice to change my mechanics and physiology, and a lot of mental monitoring and adjustment.

Changing my mind changed my breathing, and changing my breathing changed my mind. Working it from both angles brought change... faster than I would have guessed.

The golden key? Swim *your* workout, even if it's within the context of a group workout. Not the person next to you. Yours. That's how you develop a breath that works for you, not against you.

8 Breathing Drills for Swimmers

Time to find your lane. Literally. And figuratively. Here are my top eight swimming drills based on your current Breath Fitness Score to take the guesswork out of your swim-breathwork strategy.

Drill 1: Hum Before You Jump In
BFS: 53 – 100

Before you even hit the water, try humming each exhale gently for two to ten minutes. Sounds strange, but it gives you a boost of nitric oxide (a natural gas that helps blood flow), helps prepare your diaphragm, and is oddly soothing. A pro tip from Andrew Huberman would be to bias the "h" of the hum over the "m" for a bump in vagus nerve tone (functioning). [168]

Drill 2: Start Your Warm-Up Gently
BFS: 0 – 100

Most people overdo it right away. Don't. Swim slower than you think you need to and try breathing less frequently than usual – just a little less. That gives your body time to adjust before you ramp up. Some of the fastest swimmers I know are great at swimming slow.

Drill 3: Nose Breathe at the Walls (resting)
BFS: 40 – 100

Nose breathe at the wall (resting between sets). This builds CO_2 tolerance, regulates your nervous system, and encourages calm, steady recovery. I get that it will feel hard at first, but I guarantee it will get easier. And it pays dividends in and out of the pool. I know that means less talking to your lane mates, so think of it as "most of the time." As stated in the beginning, while swimming, breathe in through your mouth. Additionally, breathe out, at least partially through your nose. This way you win half the nose-breathing-game and keep water from shooting up your nose.

Drill 4: Play with Your Exhales

BFS: 60 – 100

There are a few creative ways to train how you breathe out:

- *Hum exhale:* Breathe out through your nose with a quiet hum. This builds CO_2 tolerance, diaphragm control, and nitric oxide [55-58, 169-172]

- *Trickle exhale:* Let your breath out slowly and softly through your nose. Great for subtle diaphragm work and ideal for long-distance swims where smooth efficiency beats brute strength

- *Blast exhale:* Blow out as forcefully as you can (nose and mouth) before inhaling. Great for short sprints and diaphragm strength

Drill 5: Two-Phase Pull Set

In this drill, you'll swim sets of fifty meters (two lengths of a short pool), switching between your normal breathing pattern and a slightly harder one. It's best to do this as a swim of at least two hundred meters or longer. It's even better if you use a pull buoy (the foam float you hold between your thighs) and hand paddles, so you can concentrate on your breathing and arm pull.

Your base breathing pattern is how many strokes you usually take before taking a breath. This is a rhythm you could keep up over a longer distance. For example, a beginner might use this pattern for one hundred metres, while a competitive swimmer might hold it for five hundred meters.

Your challenge breathing pattern is simply your base plus two strokes. So, if you normally breathe every three strokes, your challenge would be to breathe every five strokes.

In practice, you'll swim two laps of the pool breathing with your base pattern, then two laps breathing with your challenge pattern, and keep repeating this for the distance you've chosen. I usually recommend two hundred meters for general fitness swimmers, or three hundred meters for competitive swimmers.

Drill 6: Build Flip and Turn Power
BFS: 66 – 100

Dedicate a practice set or two to not breathing for two strokes before your turn on the wall, and two strokes after your turn. If you're not doing a flip turn, this also means not breathing during your open turn. I know, it's mean. But you get to breathe comfortably in the middle of the pool. Excellent for improving your streamline turn power in an out of the turn, maintaining focus, and building that precious CO_2 tolerance.

Drill 7: Zen 25s
BFS: 66 – 100

This is one of my favorite ways to train breath control and build calm confidence in the water. And CO_2 tolerance.

This activity is best done at the end of your swim. It's a great way to keep training and improving while giving your muscles and joints a bit of a break. Plus, it sets you up for a wildly effective cool-down. Note: this drill is designed for a short-course pool, but it works in longer pools as long as you adjust the breath holds as needed.

The idea here is "Zen" swimming: efficient strokes, just the right amount of effort, and no breathing. That's right. You take a good inhale before you push off, hold it, and you don't exhale until you get to the other side. It's all about control and precision. If you swim too fast or too slow, you'll struggle to keep it smooth.

Do four to ten of these "Zen 25s" with a ten to thirty second rest between each. Remember to nose breathe at the wall while resting.

If your pool is longer, add breaths accordingly.

If you can't make it a full length without a breath (or it feels like a heroic effort) add a breath during the lap but stick to that same pattern each time. If even that doesn't work and you find yourself adding more breaths each length, you're either too tired or just not ready for this activity. No worries. Put it on the shelf for another day.

Drill 8: Finish Strong with a Brilliant Cooldown
BFS: 0 – 100

Don't just coast through your cooldown zoned out. Swim slowly for a few minutes, steady your breath and tune in to how your body feels. Swim slower than what feels comfortable. End with ten light, low, slow nasal breaths at the wall to truly reset your system. The faster you pull yourself back to an active, controlled (not passive) parasympathetic state, the better it will go next time.

So, there you have it. Eight drills to practice when you next take your next plunge.

Whether you're chasing gold medals, better fitness, or just peace of mind, swimming can become one of the most powerful tools in your breathwork toolkit. Let it teach you.

Want to dig deeper with even more drills? I have a mini-course available: The Optimal Breathing Blueprint for Swimming. Go to breatheyourtruth.com/obbswim or scan the QR Code below.

Chapter 12:
Qi Gong and a Little Baloney

SOMETHING KEEPS PULLING ME BACK to this. I've been immersed in the biomechanics of movement and injury for all my professional life. It was that which led me to studying the breath, and then, thanks to a patient recommendation in Portland, to Qi Gong.

My passion for Qi Gong didn't start in an instant, it began as curiosity. While I've drifted from my practice at times, Qi Gong always seems to find me again. Like an old friend.

Over time, it's become an anchor for me. The more I lean in, the more I see how it opens new ways of accessing the human experience through movement, stillness, intention, and breath. Subtle. Powerful. Strangely essential.

But let's get real: Qi Gong is... bespoke. It has its share of mystique, for better or worse.
Floating hands, poetic names like *Dragon Gazes at the Moon*, and promises of energy shifts and emotional release. It's not for everyone. I get why some people find it a bit far-fetched. Still, I love it.

But stick with it, and something shifts. And no, it's not just your imagination.

If this is your first time hearing about Qi Gong, and you've got no experience, Qi Gong is a traditional Chinese practice that combines gentle movement, breathwork, and focused intention to cultivate and balance the body's life force energy. This is known as *qi* (pronounced "chee"). It's often described as a moving meditation, designed to support both physical health and emotional resilience.

Sounds beautiful, right? And it is when done well.

But things can get murky. I've heard instructors brush off a relatively common report of dizziness or nausea during practice as a good thing. "You're just purging toxins," they'll say, or "you're just shifting stagnant energy."

Maybe? But probably not exactly. It's more likely the unpleasant, and not helpful, side-effects of our old enemy: hyperventilation.

I've learned this the hard way. I've lost a few Qi Gong students to hyperventilation. They didn't kick the bucket, don't worry; they just left my class. And they left because they felt crappy during practice and thought something was wrong with them. They thought the practice was "too deep" and they had not spiritually evolved enough to hang with it. They mistook the discomfort, the foggy head, and the sudden tears as part of the process: one they weren't cut out for.

In the spirit of helping people coordinate the breath with movement, before I knew better, I inadvertently coached my Qi

Gong students into over-breathing. I didn't coach enough on the importance of subtle breathing when the load is low. I do now. As we know, over-breathing shifts your blood chemistry, traps oxygen in the bloodstream, and starves your cells of the oxygen they need. [4, 5, 7, 10, 66, 67, 69, 173-175] No wonder they felt like crap.

I wish I could have told them that the dizziness they felt wasn't enlightenment knocking. It was a biochemical traffic jam. Not spiritual progress, just a bad trip in silk pants.

And when that happens during a practice designed to regulate your nervous system and nourish your body, it's a missed opportunity.

For the most part, Qi Gong is amazing, and I've seen it work wonders with people. I've seen people tap into peace on previously unimaginable levels, and I've even heard stories of people using Qi Gong as medicine that has healed all kinds of diseases. So, this chapter isn't about trashing Qi Gong, rather, it's the opposite: it's about bringing clarity to the practice thought the lens of breath science, hopefully without losing the magic. When you understand the mechanics, chemistry, and electrical effects of your breath, Qi Gong becomes a high-impact tool for total health.

Qi Gong and the Triple M Triangle

Qi Gong can really zen you out, but it isn't just a moving meditation. When we understand it through the lens of the Triple M Triangle (Mechanics, Mix, Mind) it becomes a complete breathwork practice that covers all the bases. Let's take a closer look.

1. Mechanics – The Body's Breathability

Qi Gong helps you move better, breathe better, and feel better. Simple as that.

The slow, intentional movements open the ribcage, free the spine, and coordinate the breath with motion. It's an excellent way to improve breathing capacity and control. Your diaphragm gets to stretch, your postural muscles engage, and you create space (literally) for your breath to move. But gaining physical range is only one-third of the story.

2. Mix – The Chemistry of Breathing Right (Not Big)

Here's where a lot of well-meaning practitioners unknowingly run into trouble.

When we start paying attention to the breath, there's a natural tendency to do something with it. We breathe bigger, louder, and more often. What does that do? It drops your CO_2 levels, shifts your blood pH, and ironically reduces oxygen delivery to your cells. You know this.

But a skilled teacher will have some understanding of breath physiology and may guide you through bigger breaths at the *beginning* of practice, then gently shift you into softer, subtler breathing. The inhales should get quieter. The exhales should stretch out a little longer. And this change matters.

At that point, you're not just moving through Qi Gong. You're building a smart, efficient breath mix that boosts cellular energy, sharpens brain function, and leaves you grounded, not dizzy. [176-178]

3. Mind – The Control Panel for It All

When you match your breath with movement, and your movement with intention, you're giving your nervous system an invitation to calm down. And it listens.

That's the power of Qi Gong: it's nervous system training and breath regulation. Get the pacing right, and you'll often fall naturally into your resonant breathing frequency (think six breaths per minute) which improves heart rate variability, a huge marker for overall health.

When you slow the breath, you'll also light up the vagus nerve, helping reset and tone the entire autonomic nervous system. Calm body, clear mind.

Now, let's go even deeper.

Let's take a tour through an actual Qi Gong class and see exactly how to nourish all three pillars of the Triple M Triangle in real time. We're going to layer Mechanics, Mix, and Mind over one of the most foundational forms in Qi Gong.

The Five Element Practice

This ancient sequence is based on the five elements in traditional Chinese medicine: wood, fire, earth, metal, and water. Each element is associated with different organs, emotions, and energetic qualities. And each movement in the Five Element Practice is designed to support the corresponding system in the body, physically, energetically, and emotionally.

In the next sections, I'll guide you through each element's posture, movement, breath rhythm, and mental focus.

1. Knocking on the Door of Life (Warm-up)

Triple M Focus: Mind + Mechanics

Movement: Begin in a standing position with your feet shoulder-width apart, knees slightly bent, spine tall, and arms relaxed at your sides. Gently rotate your torso side to side, letting your arms swing freely and tap your lower back and belly. Imagine you're a pellet drum, your arms are the strings, and your hands are the little balls. Your body is the drum! Continue this movement for a couple of minutes.

Breath: Keep your breath light, natural, and through the nose. Don't try to sync the breath to the movement just yet. This is just about waking up your mind-body awareness and bringing mobility to your spine.

2. Buddha Holds Up the Earth

Element: Metal

Triple M Focus: Mechanics

Movement: Begin in the same standing position as your warmup, arms by your sides. From here, inhale as you lift your hands up (palms up) the front of your body. As they rise above your face, rotate the palms up again to face the sky and gently stretch upwards (as if you're pushing up the clouds). Exhale as you lower the arms back down, palms rotate and end at the lower abdomen, facing up. Repeat.

Breath: This is your breath *mechanics* warm-up. Breathe big on purpose. Let the inhale stretch into the belly, ribs, and collarbones. This is one of the intentional moments in the practice where you're *meant* to breathe bigger than body needs. In through the nose, out through the nose, though. It's like opening the windows before cleaning the house. We'll balance the chemistry later.

3. The Fountain

Element: Water

Triple M Focus: Mechanics + Mix + Mind

Movement: Begin standing with your feet shoulder-width apart, relaxed but alert. Arms to the sides. Inhale as you float your arms up in front of you, backs of the hands facing each other. Imagine you're drawing energy straight up the centerline, like a fountain bubbling up from the ground. At collarbone height, slowly exhale and circle the hands out and around the body, gliding outward like a gentle wave at the top of the fountain. The fingertips tracing the path of water returning to its source, and you continue to circle the hands outward and down with a comfortable exhale. The hands end facing each other at the lower abdomen and rotate out to begin again. Repeat.

Breath: In this exercise we soften and like water. Return to quiet and subtle nasal breathing. Smooth, light, and low. Feel the mechanical breath effortlessly travel from the belly up. Keeping the volume of the breath subtle (low) allows CO_2 to rise gently. Optional upgrade: hum the exhale for a few rounds to boost nitric oxide and improve circulation – biasing the "h" sound over the "m." [168][55-58, 169-172]

4. Tree Sways in the Wind

Element: Wood

Triple M Focus: Mix

Movement: Begin in a grounded standing position. Bring your hands in front of your lower abdomen, as if holding a large ball of energy (elbows rounded, shoulders relaxed, palms facing each other). At the end of an exhale, begin to turn your torso slowly to the left, letting your hips remain stable and your feet stay rooted into the ground, like the trunk of a strong tree. As you inhale, point your fingers in toward the side body and raise your left hand over the crown of the head. Imagine drawing energy up the side body, from your root to the crown. With fingers pointing in toward the crown of the head turn the body back to center. With a low breath out, circle the hands down, and back to the starting position. Do this for a few rounds on each side.

Breath: Add gentle breath holds at the top and bottom of each nasal breath. Just a couple of seconds is enough. This pause builds CO_2 tolerance and helps your body learn to stay calm with less air. It also gives you a chance to feel and experience the silence at the end of the breath (it's a cool thing).

5. Cloudy Hands

Element: Fire

Triple M Focus: Mind

Movement: Start in a horse stance: feet wider than shoulder-width apart, knees gently bent, spine tall, and shoulders relaxed. Let your arms hang loosely by your sides. Begin by raising your left hand across your chest, palm facing inward, like you're holding a big ball against the chest. At the same time, the right hand moves in front of your lower belly, palm facing toward the earth (down) As your weight naturally shifts to the left foot, allow your torso to follow slightly, softly rotating toward the side the upper hand is sweeping – left in this case. Now, switch sides: the left hand lowers and sweeps down, while the right hand rises and sweeps across the chest, palms still facing inward or down. Your weight gently shifts toward the right leg as your torso follows. Continue for several rounds to each side, allowing the movement to create a smooth figure-eight rhythm through the body.

Breath: Now we link breath and movement. Inhale as one hand sweeps left, exhale as the other sweeps right. As you get comfortable with this movement and breathing pattern, there will be a gravitational pull within your body for a five second inhale, and a five second exhale. A beautiful boost to heart rate variability. Don't forget: in through the nose, out through the nose.

6. Pebble in the Pond

Element: Earth

Triple M Focus: Mind + Mix

Movement: Bring your hands to hover in front of your lower belly, palms facing upward. As you exhale, gently rotate the hands to face the earth, and glide forward, like you're tracing ripples across a still pond. Let the movement be slow and smooth, arms extending outward in front of you without locking the elbows. As you inhale, draw your hands back in toward your body, palms turning to face up. Imagine you're gathering calm energy and bringing it home to your center. Repeat this motion fluidly, without any rush. With each repetition, you can let the exhale get a little longer, like a ripple widening and softening as it reaches the edges of the pond.

Breath: Inhale for four seconds, exhale for six. This extended out-breath through the nose activates the parasympathetic nervous system and signals your body to shift into healing mode. [9, 168, 179-182]

7. Pulling Down the Heavens (Cool down)

Triple M Focus: Mechanics + Mix + Mind

Movement: Stand tall and relaxed. Feet shoulder-width apart, knees soft, arms by your sides. Begin your inhale and slowly sweep your arms out to the sides and upward, forming a wide arc overhead. Keep your palms facing up or outward as they rise, as if you're gathering energy from above. At the top, let your palms gently turn downward to face the earth. Exhale slowly as you draw your hands down the centerline of your body, passing your forehead, chest, belly, and finally resting near the lower abdomen (just below the navel). Imagine your hands are brushing away tension, clearing stagnant energy, and guiding your attention back into your body. Repeat.

Breath: This is your custom moment. Need energy? Use a slightly longer inhale. Need calm? Stretch your exhale. Want balance? Breathe evenly. Let your breath reflect your intention. That's integration. That's mastery!

What About Purging (Forced Exhale) Activities?

The observant readers among you may have noticed that the entire sequence was accompanied by nasal breathing, and at no point did I tell you to exhale through the mouth. But I'd bet my bottom dollar that the first Qi Gong how-to video you find on the internet will showcase the words "Deep breath in through the nose, and ahhhhhh, out through the mouth."

This over-dramatic oral out-breath is also known as "purging." In the words of my friend Lee Holden, "In order to cultivate new, nourishing energy, it's important to first let go of anything that's holding us back. Whether we're feeling stressed, anxious, or emotionally burdened, Qi Gong offers practices for releasing old energy so we can create space to grow."

That's what purging is for. So yes, exhaling through the mouth has a place. For those of you familiar with Qi Gong, we're talking about activities like shaking, the "Pump," or any activity that uses a big or extended exhale. The key is using purging wisely. Timing, dosage, and recovery all matter. As will your breath fitness score.

Dosage (by Breath Fitness Score) would be:

- BFS 0 - 33 → Just 1 - 2 purging breaths
- BFS 34 - 66 → Try 5 - 10 purging breaths
- BFS 67+ → Go for 10 - 20 but always follow with gentle nose breathing

Final Word

As you can see, Qi Gong doesn't need to be cloaked in mystery or reserved for the spiritually elite. When taught with care and grounded in breath science, it becomes one of the most approachable and effective ways to train all three pillars of breath: Mechanics, Mix, and Mind.

For those of you who would like to dive deeper into this practice guided by yours truly, visit breatheyourtruth.com/qigong. There you'll find both online and in-person class information, as well as a mini-course. If you'd like to join our Qi Gong community, you'd be most welcome.

I can't recommend this stuff enough. And remember, when you do Qi Gong, you're not just doing Qi Gong. You're building a resilient nervous system. You're mastering your internal environment. And you're training your breath for the better.

Chapter 13:
Yoga: The Most Misunderstood Exercise of All

YOU YOGIS LOVE TO BREATHE. Big. Deep. Often. That's awesome… until it's not.

Because even seasoned Yoga practitioners frequently, accidentally, over-breathe. And that's a problem, especially at the beginning of class, during gentle movements, or while lying in what is a well-deserved, now ruined, Savasana. If your Ujjayi breath so forceful it could knock over a houseplant, I'm especially talking to you.

The typical yogic breathing where you're consciously inhaling and exhaling during your entire Yoga session may be blowing off more CO_2 than you're producing. This is the definition of hyperventilation. [4, 5, 10, 68, 175, 183]

That ultimately means that your Yoga practice could be throwing off your acid-base balance and sending your nervous system into fight-or-flight. You're accidentally stressing your system as opposed to soothing it. This way, you end up robbing yourself of the benefits you worked so hard for and deserve.

And if you're an instructor who's all about syncing up the asanas and the movements with deep, flowing breaths, you might be unintentionally steering your students off course.

ESPECIALLY if you've been topping it all off with a breathwork session in your Savasana. If you're getting feedback that they feel "very relaxed" but look a bit spaced out, it's a sign you've likely overdone it. Oops. I know that's not what you intended, and I know that's how you were trained during your well-meaning Yoga teacher training, but this is an epidemic much bigger than you.

So, let's fix it. The good news is that you can still breathe deeply; you can still breathe big, but in moderation – and timed strategically. You don't need to ditch tradition. I actually suspect the ancients got it right. But somewhere along the way, a few key details got lost in translation, ignored, or bull-dozed over. I don't think I'm reinventing anything, just shining a little breath-science-light on what might have been intended all along.

As a note of humility before we roll any further, I feel called to share that I'm not a yogi, and I have terrifically tight hamstrings. But I've clocked hundreds of hours on the mat, enough to deeply respect the practice. More importantly, I've worked with enough yogis to see both the common pitfalls and the powerful opportunities that come with this wonderful practice.

If we understand where things go wrong, the answers to a faster, richer, and safter path start to become clear.

5 Things You're Probably Doing Wrong (and What to Do Instead)

Breath cues in Yoga can be confusing, overly simplistic, or just plain misleading. Even with the best intentions, it's easy to fall into patterns that feel "right" but actually lead you away from a healthy practice.

Here are five of the most frequent breath-related mistakes and how to transform them into powerful points of progress.

1: Breathing BIG

Big breaths aren't always good breaths. Let's clear this up:

- Big breaths mean more volume and speed than your body actually needs
- Good breaths are those that support your body, mind, and spirit right now

Big breathing often gets praised, but it can and will work against you. That dramatic Ujjayi breath (the kind where you constrict the back of your throat but fill up your entire lung capacity) might feel powerful and controlled, but if you keep it up for an hour, you might walk out feeling like you're high. Why? You've been expelling too much CO_2 and disrupting your chemistry.

Instead:

- Use a big breath as a reset, just one or two to stretch the breathing muscles (think belly, ribs and chest) to clear lactic acid. I repeat: just ONE or TWO. Don't be greedy!
- Then, return to light, low, slow breathing through the nose

2: Breathing Deep (But Failing!)

Most yogis confuse "deep" breathing (which is healthy) with BIG breathing (which *isn't*, see point above). Let's clarify:

- Deep breathing means directing the breath down into the diaphragm, belly, and pelvic floor. It's about reaching depth, not volume
- Big breathing means pulling in more air than you need and expanding the body to pull it in

Instead:
- Inhale slowly and lightly as if you could breathe all the way down to your hips
- Let your lower belly (diaphragm) move outwards
- When you *naturally* feel the need to exhale, let it out slowly and smoothly

3: Breathing *Really* Slow

Slowing down the breath is mostly beneficial, but too much of a good thing can backfire. I've seen breathing *too* slowly, too often, drop heart rate variability (HRV) and leave practitioners feeling lethargic.

Instead:

- Find your sweet spot: 4.5 to 7.5 breaths per minute is considered the optimal range for resonant breathing. That's around five seconds for an inhale, and five seconds for an exhale. You don't need to be exact, just ballpark it. This should make up the bulk of your yoga practice, but it doesn't have to be the *whole* thing. Let it be the foundation you return to, not a rule you rigidly follow
- Use a breath pacing app to find your rhythm, but once you've got it, ditch the tech and feel the rhythm internally
- Alternate between slower, deeper breaths and natural, everyday breathing. Drop the obsession, the best you can

4: Practicing Pranayama When You Shouldn't

Pranayama (yogic breathwork) includes a lot of practices that intentionally make you over-breathe, like Breath of Fire, Three-Part Breathing, Bellows Breath, Bhastrika, and Kapalabhati. These practices are often known as "purging" practices where you intentionally get high and get rid of CO_2. (See the previous chapter for more information on purging in case you skipped it.) While these can be powerful, they're also intense and can destabilize your biochemistry and most nervous systems if overused or done incorrectly, as with any hyperventilation practice.

Instead:

- Check your Breath Fitness Score. If you're a yogi and it's below 76, focus on foundational breathing before diving into any fancy breathwork practices
- If you're ready for purging practices, use them sparingly
- Always follow intense breathwork with a grounding practice like resonant breathing or gentle nasal breathing

5: Skipping the Chill

Ever rushed out of class or jumped to the next task without soaking in that post-practice stillness? That afterglow is when your nervous system processes what just happened, integrating the benefits and allowing itself to recalibrate. Skipping it is like skipping the whole point. The work isn't just for the sake of doing, it's to spark change when you're still. Don't miss it.

Instead:

- Honor the afterglow. Whether it's a full reclined Savasana (laying down on your back relaxing for up to twenty minutes) or just a few extra minutes of stillness, take a moment to pause
- Protect those mini Savasanas throughout the practice, those relaxation pauses after a challenging pose or sequence

Ready for an Experiment?

Now that you know how to avoid the usual breathwork traps, let's look at how to level up your Yoga practice using your breath.

Before diving into any movement, close your eyes, sit tall, and simply observe the natural rhythm of your breath. There's no need to adjust or control it. Just notice where it is: high in the chest, low in the belly, shallow, or deep. This is your starting point.

Once you're tuned in, bring your focus to the lower belly and hips. Imagine your breath travelling all the way down and filling that area. The goal isn't to take a massive, dramatic breath but to explore subtle, deep breathing. Feel how the diaphragm moves as you inhale and how it gently returns as you exhale.

Now, take that deeper, quieter breath into your flow. Move through a simple sun salutation, but let the breath set the pace, not the other way around. The breath is your instructor now. Let each inhale gently lift you, each exhale ground you. Keep the breath slow, light, and low.

Once you've mastered that connection, it's time to break it. Move through another round of sun salutations, but this time, allow the breath and movement to operate independently. Let the breath stay calm and steady, even if the body is moving faster or slower than usual. This disconnection trains your nervous system to stay grounded no matter what's happening externally.

Now that you're more attuned to your breath, move into a balancing pose like tree pose. Instead of gripping or holding your breath, focus on maintaining a smooth, even flow. The aim is to find steadiness in both the body and the breath, even as you wobble or adjust.

End with Savasana. Let everything go. Feel the floor beneath you, the weight of your body, the rise and fall of your belly. This is the time to let the practice integrate. There's nothing to do, nowhere to go. Just allow yourself to breathe as your wisdom sees fit.

Final Thoughts

It's probably a good time to address a common concern. I hear this a lot:

"But David, if I'm in a class, surely I need to do what I'm told? If the teacher tells us to take big, deep breaths or do a breathwork technique and I don't do it, I'll be the odd one out. Won't the teacher feel disrespected?"

Well, here's the thing: Yoga is about tuning in, not just following along. Your breath is your own. You're the one who has to live in your body after class, not the teacher. If the breath cues don't feel right or they're taking you out of balance, you have every right to adjust. Think of it this way: if the teacher told you to hold a pose that hurt your back, would you do it just to fit in? Probably not. (Hopefully not!) So why should your breath be any different?

And it doesn't have to be a big deal. You don't need to make a scene or call out the teacher. Just subtly adjust your breathing to suit what your body needs in that moment. If the instructor says, "Big breath in," you can take a slow, steady one instead. If they're pushing heavy, dramatic Ujjayi, you can keep it light and low.

Here's a little secret: most instructors are so wrapped up in leading the class, they won't even notice what you're doing with your breath. And if they do? You're not being rude. You're being responsible. You're practicing self-regulation, which is kind of the whole point of Yoga in the first place.

Want to take your breath deeper into your Yoga practice? I've put together a thirty-minute on-demand course that explores breath-driven Yoga drills, techniques, and integration strategies, built for real bodies and real-life practice.

Head to breatheyourtruth.com/obbyoga or scan the QR code below to dive in.

Chapter 14:
Runners: Masters of Movement, Maniacs of Breathing?

RUNNERS, ABOVE ALL OTHER ATHLETES, breathe like absolute maniacs. Gasping, huffing, puffing into their chests, faces contorting with every stride like they're fleeing a bear instead of chasing a PR. But it's not entirely their fault.

Cyclists and rowers for example, are anchored to handlebars or oars, and these constraints naturally encourage breath control. But runners? Arms swinging free, legs all over the place, heads bobbing violently: it's a perfect storm for breathing chaos. And the culture doesn't help. Grit and grind are practically glamorized. Somewhere along the way, effort and over-breathing got mistaken for the same thing.

There you are, just a quarter of a mile in with your mouth gaping like a line-caught tuna. (And by the way, that over breathing is one of the top reasons runners get that dreaded side stitch later in the run.) The result? Runners have become the accidental rockstars of breathing dysfunction.

My good friend David McHenry, Physical Therapist, Strength Coach with Union Athletics Club, and Performance Coach for Nike's elite runners, dragged me into the world of running.

Through our collaboration, I've had the chance to work with collegiate athletes, Nike pros, and most recently, Under Armour's professional 800-meter team. Big thanks and a quick shoutout to Tom Brumlik, Under Armour's incredibly diligent 800-meter coach, for that opportunity.

So while running isn't my own athletic background, I've been lucky to gain deep experience from the inside. And I can tell you; there's no shortage of breathing dysfunction there.

Let's fix that.

Use Running to Train Your Breath (Not Break It)

First up, if you're a runner yourself, I'd encourage you to see running as breathwork whether you mean it to be or not. Every time you lace up and head out, you're training your breath for better or worse.

Running can be one of the best breath training tools though, if you train it on purpose. By layering in breath awareness, control, and intentional CO_2 exposure into your runs, you unlock a whole new level of performance. You become more efficient, using less oxygen to do more work. Sounds good, right? You also begin to balance your nervous system. When you stay calm early in a run, you stay strong later.

Running this way doesn't just train your muscles; it trains your chemistry. You build greater tolerance to CO_2 and lactic acid, giving your body the resilience to push further without crashing. Breath control helps manage your heart rate, which speeds up recovery and sets you up for bigger, better efforts next time.

And perhaps the most underrated benefit: mindfulness and the peace that comes with it. Nothing centers the mind quite like breath-aware movement. When your breath and stride are in sync, the noise fades. You feel steady. Grounded. Happy. Alive.

Let's explore some core running breathwork upgrades for you to try. The trick is to start simple and build as you're ready. Pick what fits, experiment with it, and grow from there.

At the end of the upgrades, you'll find a table showing how frequently and to what extent you should implement each one based on your Breath Fitness Score.

Upgrade 1: Hum Before Practice

Before you begin, try this: take a gentle nasal inhale, then hum softly on the exhale. Find a comfortable, steady pitch, it doesn't have to be perfect, and it can vary a bit based on what feels natural. This kind of soft, controlled humming has been shown to significantly boost nitric oxide, which helps oxygen get where it's needed. Bias the "H" part of the hum to get a bump on the autonomic nervous system balancing-power of the vagus nerve.

[168] I recommend starting with just a few minutes and gradually building up to ten as it feels comfortable.

Upgrade 2: Cool the Warmup

Don't rush it. Some of the fastest runners I know are masters at running slow. During warmup, start slower and breathe just a little less than you think you need, but keep it comfortable. Let yourself be surprised by how good it can feel.

Upgrade 3: Pay Attention

The simplest tool with the biggest impact: awareness. Just watching your breath improves efficiency. Seriously. If paying attention to your breathing as you run feels claustrophobic (common), hang in there. That's part of the training and it passes.

Upgrade 4: Nose Breathing

This one's pure gold: only breathe through your nose when you run. Nasal breathing trains your body to handle higher CO_2 levels, calms your nervous system, and boosts performance with less effort. It's resilience training, hidden in plain sight. [3, 7, 9, 28, 65, 135]

The problem? Most runners default to fast, shallow mouth breathing, skipping the nose's natural superpowers: filtration, humidification, and nitric oxide production. Over time, this weakens the nasal passages and makes nose breathing feel hard or even impossible. But it's not.

You weren't born a mouth breather. Most runners can retrain their anatomy with time and consistency. You might get a bit of snot coming out to say hello when you first try and nasal breathe while you run, but the nose adapts back. (Just take a tissue with you.) Nose breathing breaks the cycle of panic-mode running and rewires your system for calm, focused effort that way more efficient.

I've given this tip to dozens of runners. It hasn't failed yet. If it doesn't work for you, I want to hear about it.

Upgrade 5: Hum or Trickle Your Exhales

Hum or trickle on exhales mid-run to build diaphragm control. By trickle, I mean release the exhale as slowly as you can. This is a ninja move; it taps the entire Triple M Triangle. Humming and trickling activates the diaphragm and gently retrains your breath away from shallow chest patterns too.

Many runners, due to posture and momentum, default to upper-chest breathing. It feels easier… at first. But over time, it sidelines the diaphragm and shifts the workload to the neck, shoulders, and upper back leading to stiffness, strain, and inefficient breathing. Humming and trickling break that loop. Start with three of these and build to ten over time.

Upgrade 6: Blast Exhales

These are not for everyone but can be very effective for competitive sprints and high intensity hill repeats. These are sharp, forceful exhales that fire from the belly and rapidly draw the diaphragm in, like a bullet to the spine. The inhale? Passive. It should happen naturally after a blast exhale. This builds diaphragm coordination and strength. It sharpens breath control for the athletes among you.

Upgrade 7: Zen 100s

Let's borrow an exercise from swimmers called Zen 25s (named for one length of a short course pool). But we'll call it Zen 100s.

Pick a short stretch (about 100 meters) and run it as a "no-breather." No breathing for one hundred meters. You just take a natural breath in and hold it. Don't worry, this isn't going to make you hyperventilate. The metabolic demand makes sure your CO_2 levels don't drop. This is all about training control and efficiency.

Run too fast, and you'll blow through your reserves. Too slow, and you'll lose rhythm and control. The sweet spot is that "just right" pace for you. Repeat five to ten times during your run, with about a twenty to thirty-second rest between each. Best done at the end of your workout to refine technique, calm the system, and finish with focus.

Upgrade 8: Warm the Cooldown

Don't skip this part. Your cooldown is about training your nervous system to return to baseline. Jog or walk for ten minutes after your run. Let your breath slow. Most runners finish a workout and stay revved up, breathing too fast and too big. But with a little attention, you can rewire your recovery. This is how you teach your system to bounce back faster. Calming the breath = calming the body = more resilience next time. It's one of the simplest, most powerful ways to boost HRV, overall health, and long-term gains. [165]

As I mentioned before, all eight upgrades aren't for everyone. Let's take a look at how to apply them to your workout based on your breath fitness score.

ACTIVITY	BFS 0–33	BFS 34-66	BFS 61-100
Hum before	2 min	5 min	10 min
Cool warmup/ Warm cooldown	Yes	Yes	Yes
Pay attention	Yes	Yes	Yes
Nose breathe	Warm-up + Cool-down	50% workout	90% workout
Hum during	1 x 4 breaths	4 x 4 breaths	10 x 4 breaths
Trickle exhale	2 min	5 min	5 min
Blast exhale	1 x 10	2 x 10	3 x 10
Zen 100s	0	5	10

One additional activity is worth mentioning, even though I'm not officially including it in this program. It's called "Shark Fit," and it comes from Patrick McKeown, author of *The Oxygen Advantage* and creator of the Oxygen Advantage Method. This exercise combines hypercapnia (elevated CO_2) and hypoxia (reduced O_2), and it's designed to build serious breath efficiency and resilience under stress.

I bring it up because I think it has real value. I'm a certified advanced instructor with the Oxygen Advantage myself, that's how much I believe in it, but I'm holding it back here because it really needs individual coaching to be done safely and effectively.

If you're curious, I encourage you to read more about it in Patrick's book, *The Oxygen Advantage.*

A Note on the Difference Between Training and Competition

If you're involved in races, this part is for you. There's a real physiological and behavioral split between training and competition and understanding it can completely change how you run.

Training is where you make your deposits. You're stacking CO_2 tolerance, building neuromuscular coordination, and upgrading your metabolic efficiency. You push your chemoreceptors to stop panicking at the first hint of CO_2. You stress the nervous system, challenge the musculoskeletal system, and crucially, you recover. It's a game of adaptation: flirt with failure, then rebuild stronger.

But competition? That's when you cash in your chips. It's your savings withdrawal. You're no longer provoking the system, you're trusting it. CO_2 tolerance has already been trained; now you want just enough ventilation to keep the engine running smoothly and quickly. You're not trying to build capacity anymore. You're trying to access it.

In training, nasal breathing builds your foundation, supporting nitric oxide levels, refining mechanics, and teaching control. But in competition, the rules shift. If nasal breathing supports your effort, great. If not, let it go. Don't cling to it if it costs you power output, muscular recruitment or speed.

Years ago, a runner from the University of Oregon came back from her first 1500-meter race after several months of breath training with me.

She said, "I stayed nasal the whole time, around twelve breaths per minute."

My first thought? "Oh no. I must've forgotten to tell her it's okay to shift gears during a race."

But then she said, "It felt amazing. I ran a personal best (and I won)."

I thought it might be a fluke. But I kept hearing it from different athletes, repeatedly. Turns out, if the training is dialed in, the system doesn't just survive nasal breathing in competition: it thrives with it.

But still, here's my advice, and I mean it: when it's time to race, just run. Let the system you trained do its job. Put the time in during training though, so when race day comes, you can lean into the work you've done, the wisdom your body has stored, and the calm your mind knows by heart.

And with that… it's time to fly.

Want to go deeper? I've got more for you. I've created a 30-minute on-demand course packed with the top running drills used by professional athletes. This is for those of you who want to fine-tune your technique and unlock your best runs yet. You can check it out at breatheyourtruth.com/obbrun or just scan the QR code below to get started.

Closing Thoughts

IF YOU'VE MADE IT THIS FAR, through the myths and magic of breathwork, let me say this: I'm honored.

You've explored the breath in ways most people never do. You've unpacked its science, its subtlety, its power, and its potential risks. You've learned that breathwork isn't just about breathing more or breathing differently, it's about understanding yourself more deeply. It's about aligning your body, your chemistry, and your mind with the best version of yourself.

That's no small thing. Yes, this book is packed with fun facts, but my real hope is that it's inspired you to *practice*, not just float through the pages passively. Because once you start practicing, something shifts. You begin to see the breath for what it really is: your connection to life itself.

So, what if it's a rocky start? So, what if some days you nail it and others you fall flat? That's not failure. The breath doesn't ask for perfection. It invites you to show up, to listen, to feel what's here and respond to it healthily. To be alive in the moment.

How will you start? You've been exposed to it all: breathing while sitting, standing, walking, sleeping, exercising, swimming, lifting weights, cat-cowing, waving your "cloudy hands" wearing those flowing silk pants of yours. There's no wrong answer. Perhaps you've already started.

But if you ever find yourself forgetting, (as I do in patches where life gets tough and takes my breath away), I'd say remember to do three things: go soft, go hard, and go nowhere.

Go soft: by taking a walk outside in nature. Slow your breath down and let it go low. This is your base. Your foundation. Your most important work.

Go hard: sprinkle in the challenges. Build tolerance to nose breathing during exercise and activity. Do some breath holds. Push your CO_2 tolerance a bit. And to a lesser extent (and only if your breath fitness warrants), experiment with fancy big breathing breathwork from time-to-time.

Go nowhere: as you just sit with the breath. Sit in stillness and watch where your mind tends to travel. Notice the stories. Recognize that your mind can be trained, for better or for worse. Choose better. Your breath will reflect the mind you're shaping.

And please remember: this book was a guide, not a gospel. Let what you've learned here support your truth, not override it. You can always return to this book and revisit the content (and hey, you can even come visit me in person if you'd like to dive deeper) but your body will always be your best teacher.

Oh, and one more piece of advice, if you'd humor me. Don't forget to laugh along the way. Laughing is great for your breathing health. And as Oscar Wilde put it: "Life is too important to be taken seriously."

Wherever this work takes you, from sitting on your sofa to sprinting around a track, know that I'm cheering you on from the sidelines.

Breathe quietly. Breathe boldly. Breathe your truth.

Before you close this book…

Take a moment.

Let your shoulders settle.

Melt your jaw.

Relax your belly.

Take one gentle breath in: nose, slow, low, and steady.

Pause for a split moment.

Feel the gravity of stillness.

Then exhale comfortably, until you arrive again at a new stillness.

Feel yourself land.

Your journey is the gravity created,

by the coming, the going,

and the stillness in between.

This gravity is your anchor.

This anchor is your truth.

In just one breath, you can touch it anytime.

Touch it often.

May your breath be your guide,

your playground,

your teacher,

your refuge,

and your quiet rebellion.

- David Deppeler

Acknowledgements

First and foremost, thank you to my partner, Marcel Goot, who nudged, prodded, and lovingly pushed me to write this book. He knew the time had come long before I did. Thank you for creating space and never backing down with your support.

To my brilliant, spicy, and always-British editor, Amy White, you made this process fun and funny. Your precision made this book better. Thank you.

Thank you to Mike Long, who dove into this work with two feet and let me poke around his thought process (as well as his carbon dioxide levels with a CapnoTrainer). Your curiosity and expertise around human behavior continues to blow my mind. Thank you very much for the foreword.

To Peter Litchfield at Better Physiology, thank you for launching me down this path twenty years ago, and for your continued support with all things CapnoTrainer.

Big thanks to David McHenry, PT, DPT, Nike's Performance Coach for Elite Runners, for bombarding me with world-class athletes. You forced me to figure out what I was doing, fast. I loved every second.

And to my fellow pitta yogi - Sarahjoy Marsh of Yogajoy in Portland, OR. We've impressed and pressed each other, true to our nature. I deeply value our yearly connection points during your advanced Yoga teacher trainings. Thank you for welcoming me into your world, and for so generously supporting mine.

Thank you to Therapeutic Associates Inc, my previous employer of nearly twenty-five years, for giving Kelly Reed, Kat Burns, and me the space to experiment and develop a breathwork program from the ground up.

And finally, thank you to all the clients who have been on this journey with me. From those navigating anxiety, fatigue, and pain to those pushing for better athletic performance, thank you for showing up with honesty and commitment. We've travelled far together and learned a lot along the way. I'm deeply grateful for your trust, your willingness to do the work, and your courage to keep going.

Dr. David Deppeler is a physical therapist scientist-turned-breath whisperer helping people live how they're built to live. If you'd like more support from David and to explore his online breathing programs and community, visit breatheyourtruth.com.

Reference List

1.   Nestor, J., *Breath : the new science of a lost art*. 2020, New York: Riverhead Books. pages cm.

2.   *Cambridge dictionary of American English*. 2nd ed. 2008, Cambridge; New York: Cambridge University Press. xvi, 1104 p.

3.   Fried, R., *Breathe Well, Be Well: A Program to Relieve Stress, Anxiety, Asthma, Hypertension, Migraine, and other Disorders for Better Health*. 1991, New York: John Wiley & Sons.

4.   Fried, R., *The hyperventilation syndrome*. Biofeedback Self Regul, 1989. 14(3): p. 259-61.

5.   Fried, R., *The hyperventilation syndrome--research and clinical treatment*. J Neurol Neurosurg Psychiatry, 1988. 51(12): p. 1600-1.

6.   Fried, R., M.C. Fox, and R.M. Carlton, *Effect of diaphragmatic respiration with end-tidal CO2 biofeedback on respiration, EEG, and seizure frequency in idiopathic epilepsy*. Ann N Y Acad Sci, 1990. 602: p. 67-96.

7.   Fried, R. and J. Grimaldi, *The psychology and physiology of breathing : in behavioral medicine, clinical psychology, and psychiatry*. The Plenum series in behavioral psychophysiology and medicine. 1993, New York: Plenum Press. xxiv, 374 p.

8.   Joshi, G., et al., *Examining the clinical correlates of autism spectrum disorder in youth by ascertainment source*. J Autism Dev Disord, 2014. 44(9): p. 2117-26.

9.   Balban, M.Y., et al., *Brief structured respiration practices enhance mood and reduce physiological arousal*. Cell Rep Med, 2023. 4(1): p. 100895.

10.   Boulding, R., et al., *Dysfunctional breathing: a review of the literature and proposal for classification.* Eur Respir Rev, 2016. 25(141): p. 287-94.

11.   Courtney, R. and M. Cohen, *Investigating the claims of Konstantin Buteyko, M.D., Ph.D.: the relationship of breath holding time to end tidal CO2 and other proposed measures of dysfunctional breathing.* J Altern Complement Med, 2008. 14(2): p. 115-23.

12.   Courtney, R., K.M. Greenwood, and M. Cohen, *Relationships between measures of dysfunctional breathing in a population with concerns about their breathing.* J Bodyw Mov Ther, 2011. 15(1): p. 24-34.

13.   McKeown, P., *The oxygen advantage : the simple, scientifically proven breathing techniques for a healthier, slimmer, faster, and fitter you.* First edition. ed. 2015, New York, NY: William Morrow, an imprint of HarperCollinsPublishers. xiv, 352 pages.

14.   Kiesel, K., et al., *EXERCISE INTERVENTION FOR INDIVIDUALS WITH DYSFUNCTIONAL BREATHING: A MATCHED CONTROLLED TRIAL.* Int J Sports Phys Ther, 2020. 15(1): p. 114-125.

15.   Kiesel, K., et al., *DEVELOPMENT OF A SCREENING PROTOCOL TO IDENTIFY INDIVIDUALS WITH DYSFUNCTIONAL BREATHING.* Int J Sports Phys Ther, 2017. 12(5): p. 774-786.

16.   Rakhimov, A. *Minute Ventilation.* June 9, 2021]; Available from: https://normalbreathing.com/minute-ventilation/.

17.   Hall, J.E. and M.E. Hall, *Guyton and Hall textbook of medical physiology.* 14th edition. ed. 2021, Philadelphia, PA: Elsevier. xix, 1132 pages.

18.   Bishop, D. and B. Claudius, *Effects of induced metabolic alkalosis on prolonged intermittent-sprint performance.* Med Sci Sports Exerc, 2005. 37(5): p. 759-67.

19.   Woorons, X., et al., *Effects of a 4-week training with voluntary hypoventilation carried out at low pulmonary volumes.* Respir Physiol Neurobiol, 2008. 160(2): p. 123-30.

20.   Bentley, T. and B. Mackenzie *CO2 Tolerance and Anxiety Study.* 2020.

21.   Stanley, N.N., et al., *Evaluation of breath holding in hypercapnia as a simple clinical test of respiratory chemosensitivity.* Thorax, 1975. 30(3): p. 337-43.

22.   Zhang, L., et al., *New volumetric capnography-derived parameter: a potentially valuable tool for detecting hyperventilation during cardiopulmonary resuscitation in a porcine model.* J Thorac Dis, 2021. 13(6): p. 3467-3477.

23.   Bohr, C., K. Hasselbalch, and A. Krogh. *Concerning a Biologically Important Relationship - The Influence of the Carbon Dioxide Content of Blood on its Oxygen Binding.* 1904 [cited 2021.

24.   Shimozawa, Y., et al., *Point Prevalence of the Biomechanical Dimension of Dysfunctional Breathing Patterns Among Competitive Athletes.* The Journal of Strength & Conditioning Research, 2023. 37(2): p. 270-276.

25.   Bandyopadhyay, A. and J.E. Slaven, *Health outcomes associated with improvement in mouth breathing in children with OSA.* Sleep Breath, 2021. 25(3): p. 1635-1639.

26.   Barker, P.M., et al., *Decreased sodium ion absorption across nasal epithelium of very premature infants with respiratory distress syndrome.* J Pediatr, 1997. 130(3): p. 373-7.

27.   Basheer, B., et al., *Influence of mouth breathing on the dentofacial growth of children: a cephalometric study.* J Int Oral Health, 2014. 6(6): p. 50-5.

28. Bentley, T.G.K., et al., *Breathing Practices for Stress and Anxiety Reduction: Conceptual Framework of Implementation Guidelines Based on a Systematic Review of the Published Literature.* Brain Sciences, 2023. 13(12): p. 1612.

29. Bhaskar, L., et al., *Assessment of Cardiac Autonomic Tone Following Long Sudarshan Kriya Yoga in Art of Living Practitioners.* J Altern Complement Med, 2017. 23(9): p. 705-712.

30. Bordoni, B., et al., *The Influence of Breathing on the Central Nervous System.* Cureus, 2018. 10(6): p. e2724.

31. Alqutami, J., et al., *Dental health, halitosis and mouth breathing in 10-to-15 year old children: A potential connection.* Eur J Paediatr Dent, 2019. 20(4): p. 274-279.

32. Boyd, K.L., *A century of adenotonsillectomy's failure to fully resolve sleep-disordered breathing: mild malocclusions are maybe not so mild?* J Clin Sleep Med, 2020. 16(8): p. 1229-1230.

33. Bordoni, B. and E. Zanier, *Anatomic connections of the diaphragm: influence of respiration on the body system.* Journal of multidisciplinary healthcare, 2013: p. 281-291.

34. Dempsey, J.A., A. La Gerche, and J.H. Hull, *Is the healthy respiratory system built just right, overbuilt, or underbuilt to meet the demands imposed by exercise?* J Appl Physiol (1985), 2020. 129(6): p. 1235-1256.

35. Finta, R., et al., *Does inspiration efficiency influence the stability limits of the trunk in patients with chronic low back pain?* J Rehabil Med, 2020. 52(3): p. jrm00038.

36. Finta, R., E. Nagy, and T. Bender, *The effect of diaphragm training on lumbar stabilizer muscles: a new concept for improving segmental stability in the case of low back pain.* J Pain Res, 2018. 11: p. 3031-3045.

37. Hart, N., et al., *Evaluation of an inspiratory muscle trainer in healthy humans.* Respir Med, 2001. 95(6): p. 526-31.

38.   Hodges, P.W. and S.C. Gandevia, *Changes in intra-abdominal pressure during postural and respiratory activation of the human diaphragm.* J Appl Physiol (1985), 2000. 89(3): p. 967-76.

39.   Hodges, P.W. and S.C. Gandevia, *Activation of the human diaphragm during a repetitive postural task.* J Physiol, 2000. 522 Pt 1: p. 165-75.

40.   Hsu, S.L., et al., *Effects of core strength training on core stability.* J Phys Ther Sci, 2018. 30(8): p. 1014-1018.

41.   Key, J., *'The core': understanding it, and retraining its dysfunction.* J Bodyw Mov Ther, 2013. 17(4): p. 541-59.

42.   Kocjan, J., et al., *Network of breathing. Multifunctional role of the diaphragm: a review.* Advances in respiratory medicine, 2017. 85(4): p. 224-232.

43.   KOLAR, P., et al., *Analysis of diaphragm movement during tidal breathing and during its activation while breath holding using MRI synchronized with spirometry.* Physiol Res, 2009. 58(3): p. 383-92.

44.   Malátová, R. and P. Drevikovská, *Testing procedures for abdominal muscles using the muscle dynamometer SD02.* Proc Inst Mech Eng H, 2009. 223(8): p. 1041-8.

45.   O'Sullivan, P.B., et al., *Altered motor control strategies in subjects with sacroiliac joint pain during the active straight-leg-raise test.* Spine (Phila Pa 1976), 2002. 27(1): p. E1-8.

46.   Onders, R.P., *The diaphragm: how it affected my career and my life. The search for stability when the problem is instability.* Am J Surg, 2015. 209(3): p. 431-5.

47.   Mitka, M., *1998 NObel Prize winners are announced: three discoverers of nitric oxide activity.* JAMA, 1998. 280(19): p. 1648.

48.   Hansson, G.K., H. Jörnvall, and S.G. Lindahl, *[1998 Nobel Prize in physiology or medicine. Nitric oxide as a signal molecule in*

the cardiovascular system]. Lakartidningen, 1998. 95(43): p. 4703-8.

49.   SoRelle, R., *Nobel prize awarded to scientists for nitric oxide discoveries*. Circulation, 1998. 98(22): p. 2365-6.

50.   Bhandary, U.V., et al., *Endothelial nitric oxide synthase polymorphisms are associated with hypertension and cardiovascular disease in renal transplantation*. Nephrology (Carlton), 2008. 13(4): p. 348-55.

51.   Bhavanani, A.B., et al., *Immediate cardiovascular effects of pranava pranayama in hypertensive patients*. Indian J Physiol Pharmacol, 2012. 56(3): p. 273-8.

52.   Bian, K. and F. Murad, *Nitric oxide (NO)--biogeneration, regulation, and relevance to human diseases*. Front Biosci, 2003. 8: p. d264-78.

53.   Bennett, W.D., et al., *Effect of uridine 5'-triphosphate plus amiloride on mucociliary clearance in adult cystic fibrosis*. Am J Respir Crit Care Med, 1996. 153(6 Pt 1): p. 1796-801.

54.   Lundberg, J.O.N., et al., *High nitric oxide production in human paranasal sinuses*. Nature Medicine, 1995. 1(4): p. 370-373.

55.   Maniscalco, M., et al., *Humming-induced release of nasal nitric oxide for assessment of sinus obstruction in allergic rhinitis: pilot study*. Eur J Clin Invest, 2004. 34(8): p. 555-60.

56.   Maniscalco, M., et al., *Nasal nitric oxide measurements before and after repeated humming maneuvers*. Eur J Clin Invest, 2003. 33(12): p. 1090-4.

57.   Maniscalco, M., et al., *Assessment of nasal and sinus nitric oxide output using single-breath humming exhalations*. Eur Respir J, 2003. 22(2): p. 323-9.

58.   Weitzberg, E. and J.O. Lundberg, *Humming greatly increases nasal nitric oxide*. Am J Respir Crit Care Med, 2002. 166(2): p. 144-5.

59. Feldman, J.L. and W.A. Janczewski, *Point:Counterpoint: The parafacial respiratory group (pFRG)/pre-Botzinger complex (preBotC) is the primary site of respiratory rhythm generation in the mammal. Counterpoint: the preBötC is the primary site of respiratory rhythm generation in the mammal.* J Appl Physiol (1985), 2006. 100(6): p. 2096-7; discussion 2097-8, 2103-8.

60. Feldman, J.L. and W.A. Janczewski, *The Last Word: Point:Counterpoint authors respond to commentaries on "the parafacial respiratory group (pFRG)/pre-Botzinger complex (preBotC) is the primary site of respiratory rhythm generation in the mammal".* J Appl Physiol (1985), 2006. 101(2): p. 689.

61. Beard, A., et al., *Repeated-Sprint Training in Hypoxia in International Rugby Union Players.* Int J Sports Physiol Perform, 2019. 14(6): p. 850–854.

62. Tetzlaff, K., *Return to diving after COVID-19.* Eur J Prev Cardiol, 2022. 29(9): p. e290.

63. Tetzlaff, K., *Pulmonary Physiology and Medicine of Diving.* Semin Respir Crit Care Med, 2023. 44(5): p. 705-718.

64. Tetzlaff, K., et al., *Going to Extremes of Lung Physiology-Deep Breath-Hold Diving.* Front Physiol, 2021. 12: p. 710429.

65. Fried, R., *Integrating music in breathing training and relaxation: II. Applications.* Biofeedback Self Regul, 1990. 15(2): p. 171-7.

66. Litchfield, P.M., *CapnoLearning: Respiratory Fitness and Acid-Base Regulation.* Psychophysiology Today, 2010. 7(1): p. 6-12.

67. Courtney, R., et al., *Medically unexplained dyspnea: partly moderated by dysfunctional (thoracic dominant) breathing pattern.* J Asthma, 2011. 48(3): p. 259-65.

68. Ford, M.J., et al., *Hyperventilation, central autonomic control, and colonic tone in humans.* Gut, 1995. 37(4): p. 499-504.

69.   Laffey, J., *Hypocapnia*. New England Journal of Medicine, 2002. 347(1): p. 43-53.

70.   Feinstein, J.S., et al., *Fear and panic in humans with bilateral amygdala damage*. Nat Neurosci, 2013. 16(3): p. 270-2.

71.   Feinstein, J.S., D. Gould, and S.S. Khalsa, *Amygdala-driven apnea and the chemoreceptive origin of anxiety*. Biological Psychology, 2022. 170: p. 108305.

72.   Khalsa, S.S., et al., *Panic Anxiety in Humans with Bilateral Amygdala Lesions: Pharmacological Induction via Cardiorespiratory Interoceptive Pathways*. J Neurosci, 2016. 36(12): p. 3559-66.

73.   Litman, R., *Breathable body : transforming your world and your life, one breath at a time*. 2023, Carlsbad, California: Hay House, Inc. 272 pages.

74.   Adhana, R., et al., *The influence of the 2:1 yogic breathing technique on essential hypertension*. Indian J Physiol Pharmacol, 2013. 57(1): p. 38-44.

75.   Bellissimo, G., et al., *The Effects of Fast and Slow Yoga Breathing on Cerebral and Central Hemodynamics*. Int J Yoga, 2020. 13(3): p. 207-212.

76.   Bhavanani, A.B., Madanmohan, and Z. Sanjay, *Immediate effect of chandra nadi pranayama (left unilateral forced nostril breathing) on cardiovascular parameters in hypertensive patients*. Int J Yoga, 2012. 5(2): p. 108-11.

77.   Bhavanani, A.B., et al., *Differential effects of uninostril and alternate nostril pranayamas on cardiovascular parameters and reaction time*. Int J Yoga, 2014. 7(1): p. 60-5.

78.   Wikipedia. *Dantien*. 2025 [cited 2025 June 28, 2025]; Dantiens as energy centers]. Available from: https://en.wikipedia.org/wiki/Dantian.

79.   Rückert-Eheberg, I.M., et al., *Respiratory rate and its associations with disease and lifestyle factors in the general*

population - results from the KORA-FF4 study. PLoS One, 2025. 20(3): p. e0318502.

80. Lucini, D., et al., *Correlation between baroreflex gain and 24-h indices of heart rate variability.* J Hypertens, 2002. 20(8): p. 1625-31.

81. Divine, M., *The way of the SEAL : think like an elite warrior to lead and succeed.* 2015, New York: Reader's Digest Association, Inc. xiii, 240 pages.

82. Kabat-Zinn, J., *Full catastrophe living : using the wisdom of your body and mind to face stress, pain, and illness.* Revised and updated edition. ed. 2013, New York: Bantam Books trade paperback. xlv, 650 pages.

83. Winkle, M.J. and A. Sankari, *Respiratory Muscle Strength Training*, in *StatPearls.* 2025: Treasure Island (FL).

84. Prem, V., R.C. Sahoo, and P. Adhikari, *Comparison of the effects of Buteyko and pranayama breathing techniques on quality of life in patients with asthma—a randomized controlled trial.* Clinical rehabilitation, 2013. 27(2): p. 133-141.

85. Cooper, S., et al., *Effect of two breathing exercises (Buteyko and pranayama) in asthma: a randomised controlled trial.* Thorax, 2003. 58(8): p. 674-9.

86. Beard, A., et al., *Upper-body repeated-sprint training in hypoxia in international rugby union players.* Eur J Sport Sci, 2019. 19(9): p. 1175-1183.

87. Bixler, E.O., et al., *Prevalence of sleep disorders in the Los Angeles metropolitan area.* Am J Psychiatry, 1979. 136(10): p. 1257-62.

88. Brechbuhl, C., et al., *Effects of Repeated-Sprint Training in Hypoxia on Tennis-Specific Performance in Well-Trained Players.* Sports Med Int Open, 2018. 2(5): p. E123-E132.

89. Brocherie, F., G.P. Millet, and O. Girard, *Psychophysiological Responses to Repeated-Sprint Training in Normobaric Hypoxia*

and Normoxia. Int J Sports Physiol Perform, 2017. 12(1): p. 115-123.

90.   Camacho-Cardenosa, M., et al., *Repeated-sprint training under cyclic hypoxia improves body composition in healthy women.* J Sports Med Phys Fitness, 2019. 59(10): p. 1700-1708.

91.   Fornasier-Santos, C., G.P. Millet, and X. Woorons, *Repeated-sprint training in hypoxia induced by voluntary hypoventilation improves running repeated-sprint ability in rugby players.* Eur J Sport Sci, 2018. 18(4): p. 504-512.

92.   Hamlin, M.J., et al., *Hypoxic Repeat Sprint Training Improves Rugby Player's Repeated Sprint but Not Endurance Performance.* Front Physiol, 2017. 8: p. 24.

93.   Kasai, N., et al., *Effect of training in hypoxia on repeated sprint performance in female athletes.* Springerplus, 2015. 4: p. 310.

94.   Lapointe, J., et al., *Impact of Hypoventilation Training on Muscle Oxygenation, Myoelectrical Changes, Systemic [K.* Front Sports Act Living, 2020. 2: p. 29.

95.   Trincat, L., X. Woorons, and G.P. Millet, *Repeated-Sprint Training in Hypoxia Induced by Voluntary Hypoventilation in Swimming.* Int J Sports Physiol Perform, 2017. 12(3): p. 329-335.

96.   Serebrovska, T.V., Z.O. Serebrovska, and E. Egorov, *Fitness and therapeutic potential of intermittent hypoxia training: a matter of dose.* Fiziol Zh, 2016. 62(3): p. 78-91.

97.   Pramkratok, W., T. Songsupap, and T. Yimlamai, *Repeated sprint training under hypoxia improves aerobic performance and repeated sprint ability by enhancing muscle deoxygenation and markers of angiogenesis in rugby sevens.* Eur J Appl Physiol, 2022. 122(3): p. 611-622.

98.   McKeown, P., *The Breathing Cure. Exercises to Develop New Breathing Habits for a Healthier, Happier and Longer Life.* 2021: OxyAt Books.

99.   Ivanova, D., H. Nihrizov, and O. Zhekov, *The Very Beginning*, in *Human Contact With the Underwater World*. 1999, Think Quest.

100.   Shavanani, A. and K. Udupa, *Acute effect of Mukh bhastrika (a yogic bellows type breathing) on reaction time*. Indian journal of physiology and pharmacology, 2003. 47: p. 297-300.

101.   Bhavanani, A.B., M. Ramanathan, and H. Kt, *SHORT COMMUNICATION IMMEDIATE EFFECT OF MUKHA BHASTRIKA (A BELLOWS TYPE PRANAYAMA) ON REACTION TIME IN MENTALLY CHALLENGED ADOLESCENTS.* Setting editorial goals.... 2012. 56(2): p. 174.

102.   Bhajan, *Rebirthing : breath-vitality-strength : Kundalini Yoga as taught by Yogi Bhajan*. 2011, Santa Cruz, New Mexico: Kudalini Research Institute. xii, 450 pages.

103.   Kozhevnikov, M., et al., *Neurocognitive and somatic components of temperature increases during g-tummo meditation: legend and reality*. PLoS One, 2013. 8(3): p. e58244.

104.   Benson, H., et al., *Body temperature changes during the practice of g Tum-mo yoga*. Nature, 1982. 295(5846): p. 234-6.

105.   Hof, W. and K. De Jong, *The Way of the Iceman*. 2016, Little Canada, MN: Dragon Door Publications, Inc.

106.   Hof, W., *The Wim Hof method : activate your full human potential*. 2020, Sounds True,: Boulder, CO. p. 1 online resource.

107.   Kox, M., et al., *Cytokine Levels in Critically Ill Patients With COVID-19 and Other Conditions*. JAMA, 2020.

108.   Kox, M., et al., *Voluntary activation of the sympathetic nervous system and attenuation of the innate immune response in humans*. 2014, PNAS: Nijmegen, Het Nederland.

109.   Houtman, A., et al., *Endocrine and Immune Systems*, in *Biology Now*. 2015, W. W. Norton & Company. p. 388–405.

110. Carney, S., *The Iceman Cometh*. 2011.

111. Carney, S., *What doesn't kill us : how freezing water, extreme altitude, and environmental conditioning will renew our lost evolutionary strength*. 2017, New York, NY: Rodale. xxxii, 240 pages, 16 unnumbered pages of plates.

112. Tijmstra, F. and L. Bomers. *Iceman onder vuur" [Iceman' under fire] (in Dutch)*. 2016; Available from: https://eenvandaag.avrotros.nl/item/iceman-onder-vuur/.

113. Duin, R., *Iceman oefening eist opnieuw leven [Iceman exercise claims a new life]*. 2016, Het Parool (in Dutch).

114. *Heal Yourself with The Ice Shaman, Wim Hof & Russell Brand*, in https://www.youtube.com/watch?v=JPPlicAEFec. 2019, YouTube.

115. Janakiramaiah, N., et al., *Antidepressant efficacy of Sudarshan Kriya Yoga (SKY) in melancholia: a randomized comparison with electroconvulsive therapy (ECT) and imipramine*. J Affect Disord, 2000. 57(1-3): p. 255-9.

116. Hamilton-West, K., T. Pellatt-Higgins, and F. Sharief, *Evaluation of a Sudarshan Kriya Yoga (SKY) based breath intervention for patients with mild-to-moderate depression and anxiety disorders*. Prim Health Care Res Dev, 2019. 20: p. e73.

117. Mathersul, D.C., et al., *Study protocol for a non-inferiority randomised controlled trial of SKY breathing meditation versus cognitive processing therapy for PTSD among veterans*. BMJ Open, 2019. 9(4): p. e027150.

118. Toschi-Dias, E., et al., *Sudarshan Kriya Yoga improves cardiac autonomic control in patients with anxiety-depression disorders*. J Affect Disord, 2017. 214: p. 74-80.

119. Zope, S.A. and R.A. Zope, *Sudarshan kriya yoga: Breathing for health*. Int J Yoga, 2013. 6(1): p. 4-10.

120. Brown, R.P. and P.L. Gerbarg, *Sudarshan Kriya Yogic breathing in the treatment of stress, anxiety, and depression. Part II--clinical applications and guidelines.* J Altern Complement Med, 2005. 11(4): p. 711-7.

121. Bandura, A., *The anatomy of stages of change.* Am J Health Promot, 1997. 12(1): p. 8-10.

122. Bandura, A., et al., *Multifaceted impact of self-efficacy beliefs on academic functioning.* Child Dev, 1996. 67(3): p. 1206-22.

123. Fangmeyer, S.K., C.D. Badger, and P.G. Thakkar, *Nocturnal mouth-taping and social media: A scoping review of the evidence.* Am J Otolaryngol, 2025. 46(1): p. 104545.

124. Cooper, S., et al., *Effect of mouth taping at night on asthma control--a randomised single-blind crossover study.* Respir Med, 2009. 103(6): p. 813-9.

125. Lee, D.W., J.G. Kim, and Y.M. Yang, *Influence of mouth breathing on atopic dermatitis risk and oral health in children: A population-based cross-sectional study.* J Dent Sci, 2021. 16(1): p. 178-185.

126. Lee, K.J., et al., *EEG signals during mouth breathing in a working memory task.* Int J Neurosci, 2020. 130(5): p. 425-434.

127. Lee, Y.C., et al., *The Impact of Mouth-Taping in Mouth-Breathers with Mild Obstructive Sleep Apnea: A Preliminary Study.* Healthcare (Basel), 2022. 10(9).

128. Labarca, G., et al., *Mouth Closing to Improve the Efficacy of Mandibular Advancement Devices in Sleep Apnea.* Ann Am Thorac Soc, 2022. 19(7): p. 1185-1192.

129. Bajer, B., et al., *Exercise associated hormonal signals as powerful determinants of an effective fat mass loss.* Endocr Regul, 2015. 49(3): p. 151-63.

130. Calapai, M., et al., *Effects of Physical Exercise and Motor Activity on Depression and Anxiety in Post-Mastectomy Pain Syndrome.* Life (Basel), 2024. 14(1).

131. Chan, J.S.M., et al., *Qigong exercise for chronic fatigue syndrome.* Int Rev Neurobiol, 2019. 147: p. 121-153.

132. Estrada, C., et al., *Voluntary exercise reduces plasma cortisol levels and improves transitory memory impairment in young and aged Octodon degus.* Behav Brain Res, 2019. 373: p. 112066.

133. Mahalakshmi, B., et al., *Possible Neuroprotective Mechanisms of Physical Exercise in Neurodegeneration.* Int J Mol Sci, 2020. 21(16).

134. Vollert, C., et al., *Exercise prevents sleep deprivation-associated anxiety-like behavior in rats: potential role of oxidative stress mechanisms.* Behav Brain Res, 2011. 224(2): p. 233-40.

135. Baraniuk, J.N. and S.J. Merck, *Nasal reflexes: implications for exercise, breathing, and sex.* Current allergy and asthma reports, 2008. 8(2): p. 147-153.

136. Cai, Y., A.N. Goldberg, and J.L. Chang, *The nose and nasal breathing in sleep apnea.* Otolaryngologic Clinics of North America, 2020. 53(3): p. 385-395.

137. Gilliam, K., *Benefits of Nasal Breathing.* 2020.

138. Jella, S.A. and D.S. Shannahoff-Khalsa, *The effects of unilateral forced nostril breathing on cognitive performance.* International Journal of Neuroscience, 1993. 73(1-2): p. 61-68.

139. Jung, J.-Y. and C.-K. Kang. *Investigation on the effect of oral breathing on cognitive activity using functional brain imaging.* in *Healthcare.* 2021. MDPI.

140. Marshall, R.S., et al., *Exploring the Benefits of Unilateral Nostril Breathing Practice Post-Stroke: Attention, Language, Spatial Abilities, Depression, and Anxiety.* The Journal of

Alternative and Complementary Medicine, 2014. 20(3): p. 185-194.

141. Marshall, R.S., et al., *Unilateral Forced Nostril Breathing and Aphasia—Exploring Unilateral Forced Nostril Breathing as an Adjunct to Aphasia Treatment: A Case Series.* The Journal of Alternative and Complementary Medicine, 2015. 21(2): p. 91-99.

142. Nair, S., *Nasal breathing exercise and its effect on symptoms of allergic rhinitis.* Indian Journal of Otolaryngology and Head & Neck Surgery, 2012. 64: p. 172-176.

143. Örün, D., S. Karaca, and Ş. Arıkan, *The effect of breathing exercise on stress hormones.* 2022.

144. Shturman-Ellstein, R., et al., *The beneficial effect of nasal breathing on exercise-induced bronchoconstriction.* American Review of Respiratory Disease, 1978. 118(1): p. 65-73.

145. Zelano, C., et al., *Nasal Respiration Entrains Human Limbic Oscillations and Modulates Cognitive Function.* J Neurosci, 2016. 36(49): p. 12448-12467.

146. Garg, R., et al., *Effect of Left, Right and Alternate Nostril Breathing on Verbal and Spatial Memory.* J Clin Diagn Res, 2016. 10(2): p. CC01-3.

147. Ismail, A.M.A., H. Saif, and M.M. Taha, *Effect of alternate nostril breathing exercise on autonomic functions, ocular hypertension, and quality of life in elderly with systemic hypertension and high-tension primary open-angle glaucoma.* Geriatr Nurs, 2023. 52: p. 91-97.

148. Hakked, C.S., R. Balakrishnan, and M.N. Krishnamurthy, *Yogic breathing practices improve lung functions of competitive young swimmers.* Journal of Ayurveda and Integrative Medicine, 2017. 8(2): p. 99-104.

149. Kalaivani, S., M.J. Kumari, and G.K. Pal, *Effect of alternate nostril breathing exercise on blood pressure, heart rate, and rate*

pressure product among patients with hypertension in JIPMER, Puducherry. J Educ Health Promot, 2019. 8: p. 145.

150.   Kamath, A., R.P. Urval, and A.K. Shenoy, *Effect of Alternate Nostril Breathing Exercise on Experimentally Induced Anxiety in Healthy Volunteers Using the Simulated Public Speaking Model: A Randomized Controlled Pilot Study.* Biomed Res Int, 2017. 2017: p. 2450670.

151.   Mohanty, S. and A.A. Saoji, *Comments on "Alternate Nostril Breathing at Different Rates and Its Influence on Heart Rate Variability in Non Practitioners of Yoga".* J Clin Diagn Res, 2016. 10(7): p. CL01.

152.   Pandya, J., et al., *A Pilot Study on the Effect of Alternate Nostril Breathing and Foot Reflexology on Intraocular Pressure in Ocular Hypertension.* J Altern Complement Med, 2019. 25(8): p. 824-826.

153.   Shannahoff-khalsa, D.S. and B. Kennedy, *The Effects of Unilateral Forced Nostril Breathing on the Heart.* International Journal of Neuroscience, 1993. 73(1-2): p. 47-60.

154.   Sinha, A.N., D. Deepak, and V.S. Gusain, *Assessment of the effects of pranayama/ alternate nostril breathing on the parasympathetic nervous system in young adults.* J Clin Diagn Res, 2013. 7(5): p. 821-3.

155.   Telles, S., R. Nagarathna, and H.R. Nagendra, *Breathing through a particular nostril can alter metabolism and autonomic activities.* Indian J Physiol Pharmacol, 1994. 38(2): p. 133-7.

156.   Telles, S., R. Nagarathna, and H.R. Nagendra, *Physiological Measures of Right Nostril Breathing.* The Journal of Alternative and Complementary Medicine, 1996. 2(4): p. 479-484.

157.   Aljuraifani, R., et al., *Activity of Deep and Superficial Pelvic Floor Muscles in Women in Response to Different Verbal Instructions: A Preliminary Investigation Using a Novel*

Electromyography Electrode. J Sex Med, 2019. 16(5): p. 673-679.

158. Aljuraifani, R., et al., *Task-specific differences in respiration-related activation of deep and superficial pelvic floor muscles.* J Appl Physiol (1985), 2019. 126(5): p. 1343-1351.

159. Hodges, P.W., et al., *Coexistence of stability and mobility in postural control: evidence from postural compensation for respiration.* Exp Brain Res, 2002. 144(3): p. 293-302.

160. Hodges, P.W., R. Sapsford, and L.H. Pengel, *Postural and respiratory functions of the pelvic floor muscles.* Neurourol Urodyn, 2007. 26(3): p. 362-71.

161. Smith, M.D., A. Russell, and P.W. Hodges, *Disorders of breathing and continence have a stronger association with back pain than obesity and physical activity.* Aust J Physiother, 2006. 52(1): p. 11-6.

162. Smith, M., M.W. Coppieters, and P.W. Hodges, *Effect of experimentally induced low back pain on postural sway with breathing.* Exp Brain Res, 2005. 166(1): p. 109-17.

163. Behm, D.G., et al., *Effectiveness of Traditional Strength vs. Power Training on Muscle Strength, Power and Speed with Youth: A Systematic Review and Meta-Analysis.* Front Physiol, 2017. 8: p. 423.

164. Steffen, P.R., et al., *The Impact of Resonance Frequency Breathing on Measures of Heart Rate Variability, Blood Pressure, and Mood.* Frontiers in Public Health, 2017. Volume 5 - 2017.

165. Van Hooren, B. and J.M. Peake, *Do We Need a Cool-Down After Exercise? A Narrative Review of the Psychophysiological Effects and the Effects on Performance, Injuries and the Long-Term Adaptive Response.* Sports Med, 2018. 48(7): p. 1575-1595.

166. Anderson, G. and E.C. Rhodes, *Relationship between blood lactate and excess CO2 in elite cyclists.* Journal of sports sciences, 1991. 9: p. 173-81.

167. Beaver, W.L., K. Wasserman, and B.J. Whipp, *A new method for detecting anaerobic threshold by gas exchange.* Journal of Applied Physiology, 1986. 60(6): p. 2020-2027.

168. Huberman, A., *Huberman Lab*, in *Control Your Vagus Nerve to Improve Mood, Alertness & Neuroplasticity*, A. Huberman, Editor. 2025.

169. De Winter–de Groot, K.M. and C.K. Van Der Ent, *Measurement of nasal nitric oxide: evaluation of six different sampling methods.* European Journal of Clinical Investigation, 2009. 39(1): p. 72-77.

170. Eby, G.A., *Strong humming for one hour daily to terminate chronic rhinosinusitis in four days: A case report and hypothesis for action by stimulation of endogenous nasal nitric oxide production.* Medical Hypotheses, 2006. 66(4): p. 851-854.

171. Maniscalco, M., G. Pelaia, and M. Sofia, *Exhaled nasal nitric oxide during humming: potential clinical tool in sinonasal disease?* Biomark Med, 2013. 7(2): p. 261-6.

172. Manscalco, M., *Humming, Nitric Oxide and Paranasal Sinus Ventilation*, in *Department of Physiology and Pharmacology*. 2006, Karolinska Institutet: Stockholm. p. 51.

173. Jones M, H.A., Marston L, O'Connell NE, *Breathing exercises for dysfunctional breathing/hyperventilation syndrome in adults.* Cochrane Database of Systematic Review, 2013(5).

174. van Doorn, P., H. Folgering, and P. Colla, *Control of the end-tidal PCO2 in the hyperventilation syndrome: effects of biofeedback and breathing instructions compared.* Bull Eur Physiopathol Respir, 1982. 18(6): p. 829-36.

175. Lum, L.C., *Hyperventilation syndromes in medicine and psychiatry: a review.* J R Soc Med, 1987. 80(4): p. 229-31.

176. Leung, K.-C.W., et al., *Mind-Body Health Benefits of Traditional Chinese Qigong on Women: A Systematic Review of Randomized Controlled Trials.* Evidence-Based Complementary and Alternative Medicine, 2021. 2021(1): p. 7443498.

177. Singsanan, S., et al., *Qigong Training Effects on Brain-Derived Neurotrophic Factor and Cognitive Functions in Sedentary Middle-Aged and Elderly Females With Type 2 Diabetes.* Women in Sport and Physical Activity Journal, 2024. 32(1): p. wspaj.2024-0041.

178. Sousa, M.d.L.R.d., M.I.L. Montebello, and É. Johnson, *Benefits of Qigong: a 3-Months Online Course.* Perspect Integr Med, 2025. 4(1): p. 57-61.

179. Bae, D., et al., *Increased exhalation to inhalation ratio during breathing enhances high-frequency heart rate variability in healthy adults.* Psychophysiology, 2021. 58(11): p. e13905.

180. Komori, T., *The relaxation effect of prolonged expiratory breathing.* Ment Illn, 2018. 10(1): p. 7669.

181. Magnon, V., F. Dutheil, and G.T. Vallet, *Benefits from one session of deep and slow breathing on vagal tone and anxiety in young and older adults.* Sci Rep, 2021. 11(1): p. 19267.

182. Telles, S., et al., *Vagally Mediated Heart Rate Variability and Mood States in Patients with Chronic Pain Receiving Prolonged Expiration Regulated Breathing: A Randomized Controlled Trial.* Appl Psychophysiol Biofeedback, 2024. 49(4): p. 665-675.

183. Lum, L., *Hyperventilation Syndromes.* 1994.

www.ingramcontent.com/pod-product-compliance
Lightning Source LLC
Chambersburg PA
CBHW062050270326
41931CB00013B/3019